T0205435

Biopsy Pathology of Muscle

BIOPSY PATHOLOGY SERIES

General Editors

Professor Leonard S. Gottlieb, M.D., M.P.H.
Mallory Institute of Pathology,
Boston, U.S.A.

Professor A. Munro Neville, M.D., Ph.D., M.R.C. Path.
Ludwig Institute for Cancer Research,
Sutton, U.K.

Professor F. Walker, M.D., Ph.D.
Department of Pathology,
University of Leicester, U.K.

Biopsy Pathology of Muscle

MICHAEL SWASH
M.D. (London), F.R.C.P. (London), M.R.C. Path.
Consultant Neurologist, The London Hospital
and St Mark's Hospital, London,
and Senior Lecturer in Neuropathology,
The London Hospital Medical College, London

and

MARTIN S. SCHWARTZ
M.D. (Maryland)
Consultant Clinical Neurophysiologist
St George's Hospital (Atkinson Morley's Hospital) London

SPRINGER-SCIENCE+BUSINESS MEDIA, B.V.

© *1984 M. Swash and M. S. Schwartz*
Originally published by Chapman and Hall in 1984
Softcover reprint of the hardcover 1st edition 1984

Phototypeset by
Wyvern Typesetting Ltd, Bristol

ISBN 978-0-412-24420-9

British Library Cataloguing in Publication Data
Swash, Michael
   Biopsy pathology of muscle. – (Biopsy pathology
   series)
   1. Muscles – Diseases   2. Muscle
   I. Title   II. Schwartz, Martin S.
   III. Series
   616.7'407   RC925.7

   ISBN 978-0-412-24420-9   ISBN 978-1-4899-3402-4 (eBook)
   DOI 10.1007/978-1-4899-3402-4

Contents

vi   Contents

Preface

During the last 20 years the development of enzyme histochemical techniques has contributed greatly to knowledge of muscle pathology. However, these and other new methods, such as electron microscopy and immunocytochemistry, have only relatively recently become generally available for routine use in histopathology. Muscle biopsy is a long-established technique in clinical practice, having been introduced by Duchenne in 1868 (*Arch. Gen. Med.*, **11**, 5–179). However, the needle method used by Duchenne was not generally adopted, although Shank and Hoagland described a similar technique in 1943 (*Science*, **98**, 592). During this time muscle biopsies required a surgical procedure and this was a considerable disincentive to their use. It was not until Bergstrom (1962; *Scand. J. Clin. Lab. Invest.*, **14**, Suppl. 68) and Edwards (1971; *Lancet*, **ii**, 593–6) developed a simple biopsy needle suitable for muscle work in connection with exercise physiology that the advantages of needle muscle biopsies came to be appreciated. Since then, muscle biopsies have become a relatively minor procedure. This has led to the increasing use of muscle biopsy in clinical practice, both for diagnosis and for assessing progress in repeated biopsies during the course of a disorder and its treatment. The full range of enzyme histochemical and ultrastructural histological techniques can be applied to these small biopsies and many of the older histological staining methods can also be used.

This book is intended to serve as a practical guide in muscle pathology, particularly for histopathologists, and for those in training. As enzyme histochemistry has become more widely available, formalin-fixed methods, with their inherent limitations, have become less frequently used in muscle biopsy work, and there is a thus a need for a short but complete account of muscle biopsy pathology. In this book emphasis is placed on those features which are of specific diagnostic value, or which reflect changes occurring during treatment, as in polymyositis, or at different stages of neuromuscular disorders. Electron microscopy is largely a research tool and ultrastructural features are discussed only when they are relevant to the investigation of particular disorders. Similarly, although quantitative methods are applicable to muscle biopsy pathology, microcomputer-based measurements are not generally available. Nonetheless, simple and accurate measurement can be made without technical aids of this sort and these are described. We have tried to illustrate the major problems likely to be encountered in all but the most specialized referral centres, and have provided sufficient references to guide our readers in any further exploration of the literature they may wish to undertake. A description of the clinical and physiological features of neuromuscular disorders is available in our earlier book *Neuromuscular Diseases: A Practical Approach to Diagnosis and Management*.

No book can be written without help from colleagues. We thank particularly Dr David Pollock, who kindly reviewed our account of muscle tumours as revealed by muscle biopsy, and helped with the illustrations for this chapter. Mr Ivor Northey and Mr Tim Bushnell in the department of medical photography of the Institute of Pathology at The London Hospital Medical College kindly prepared the illustrations. The work which has led to the preparation of this book has been supported, at least in part, by The London Hospital Special Trustees, The Wellcome Trust, The Medical Research Council and The London Hospital Medical College, and we gratefully acknowledge this support. A number of the illustrations are taken from our previous publications in various journals and these are reproduced here, with permission, as follows: Fig. 2.7, *Neurology (Minneapolis)*; Figs 2.13, 4.12, 7.3, 7.5 and 8.4, *Journal of Neurology, Neurosurgery and Psychiatry*; Fig. 3.5a, b, *Journal of Anatomy*; Figs 4.12c, 6.17 and 8.4, *Brain*; Figs 4.3 and 8.14, *Muscle and Nerve*; Figs 4.6, 4.7, 5.7, 5.8, 5.13, 7.1, 7.8, 8.9 and 9.4 are reproduced from our book, *Neuromuscular Diseases: A Practical Approach to Diagnosis and Management*, Springer-Verlag, Berlin, Heidelberg, New York (1981) (316 pp.).

M. Swash
The London Hospital, E1

M. S. Schwartz
St George's Hospital, SW17

1 Introduction

1.1 General features of muscle

The differentiation of muscle into red and white types is a feature of all vertebrates and, indeed, of chordates. Red muscles are slow-contracting and specialized for postural activity. They contain plentiful lipid droplets and glycogen granules and sparse mitochondria. White muscles, on the other hand, are faster contracting, suitable for short bursts of intense activity, but fatigue rapidly. They contain few lipid droplets, but plentiful mitochondria. In man these fibre types are not found exclusively in individual muscles but occur in a random distribution in all muscles. Although these two types of muscle fibre can be recognized in haematoxylin and eosin preparations of transverse sections of paraffin-embedded muscle, they can be more easily identified by the reciprocal relationship of their content of oxidative and non-oxidative enzymes (see Table 2.3). The red fibres react strongly for oxidative enzymes, e.g. succinic dehydrogenase, and are designated *Type 1 fibres*, and the white fibres react strongly for non-oxidative enzymes, e.g. myophosphorylase, and are designated *Type 2 fibres* (Dubowitz and Pearse, 1960). In cross section these two fibre types are arranged in a random mosaic pattern within muscle fascicles.

1.2 The motor unit

Each muscle fibre is innervated by a single nerve fibre, which almost invariably terminates in a single motor end-plate. The functional unit in muscle, termed the motor unit by Sherrington, consists of a single anterior horn cell situated in the grey matter of the spinal cord, the motor axon derived from this cell, and its terminal branches, innervating a number of muscle fibres. The muscle fibres making up any individual motor unit are distributed through up to 30% of the cross-sectional area of a muscle (Fig. 1.1), in several fascicles. The fibres of one motor unit are therefore intermingled with other muscle fibres belonging to other motor

1

(a)

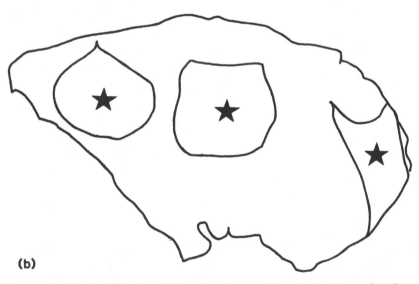

(b)

Fig. 1.1 (a) The muscle fibres belonging to a single motor unit are distributed quasi-randomly through part of the muscle. This drawing of the cross-sectional plane of a cat soleus muscle is taken from the work of Edstrom and Kugelberg (1968). The motor unit was identified by glycogen depletion after supramaximal stimulation of a single efferent nerve fibre in the appropriate ventral root. (b) Drawing of the territories of three separate motor units in the cat soleus (after Edstrom and Kugelberg, 1968).

units (Edstrom and Kugelberg, 1968; Brandstater and Lambert, 1973). The individual motor units cannot be recognized in specimens of muscle without special physiological/pathological correlation techniques.

Muscle fascicles (Fig. 1.2) are separated from each other by connective tissue which itself contains neurovascular bundles. Muscle spindles are situated in close association with these neurovascular bundles. The fascicular pattern of individual muscles varies. The length of muscle fibres in different muscles varies greatly, from a few millimeters to as much as 40 cm. Within a fascicle the muscle fibres are arranged in parallel, but individual fascicles are not usually arranged in the plane of the long axis of a muscle, but in a bipennate distribution inserting into a centrally situated tendinous plane. This arrangement may or may not be symmetrical, and there is great variability between different muscles. Golgi tendon organs are found in the major tendinous insertions and origins of muscles. The nerve supplying a muscle usually enters it, with its accompanying blood vessels, near the mid-point of the muscle.

The pathological features of diseases of muscle are determined by the disease process itself, by the intrinsic properties of muscle and by the close structural/functional relationship of muscle and its nerve supply. Thus diseases of muscle are broadly classified into *myopathies*, in which the disorder primarily affects the muscle fibres, and *neurogenic disorders*, in which muscular abnormalities result from disturbance of the innervation. By historical convention certain inherited myopathies are classified as *muscular dystrophies*, a term which implies a progressive course with marked change in the normal structure of the muscles.

1.3 Classification of neuromuscular disorders

There are a large number of different disorders in which muscle may be affected but, in the majority of these, muscle biopsy is not a useful investigation since it does not provide specific diagnostic information, and a diagnosis can be obtained more easily by other methods. For example, peripheral neuropathies, in which marked abnormalities occur in affected muscle, are usually diagnosed by clinical and electrophysiological techniques, and occasionally by nerve biopsy. In addition, many of the disorders noted in comprehensive classifications of neuromuscular disorders are extremely rare. The classification given here (Table 1.1) includes those disorders likely to be encountered in the pathological laboratory. A more complete classification is available (Walton and Gardner-Medwin, 1981). The most common condition in which muscle biopsy is likely to be performed is polymyositis, but this is not the commonest neuromuscular disorder; for example diabetic polyneuropathy is far more frequent.

Fig. 1.2 (a) × 140; NADH. Normal muscle. A muscle spindle is seen in the interfascicular plane at the junction of several fascicles in the centre of the illustration, close to a small intramuscular nerve and a blood vessel – the neurovascular bundle. Two fibre types can be identified in the extrafusal muscle fibres; the intrafusal muscle fibres are very small and react intensely in this technique. (b) × 350; HE. Normal muscle spindle in a muscle biopsy from an infant. The intrafusal and extrafusal muscle fibres are approximately equal in size.

Table 1.1 A classification of neuromuscular disorders (modified from Swash and Schwartz, 1981)

MYOPATHIC DISORDERS

1. *Inflammatory myopathies*
   (a) *Idiopathic*
       Polymyositis
       Dermatomyositis
       Childhood dermatomyositis
       Polymyositis and dermatomyositis associated with carcinoma
       Polymyositis and dermatomyositis associated with collagen–vascular disease
       Granulomatous polymyositis (sarcoidosis)
       Eosinophilic polymyositis

   (b) *Infections*
       Viral
       Bacterial
       Infestations

2. *Drug-induced myopathies*

3. *Endocrine myopathies*
       Thyroid myopathies
       Osteomalacia and parathyroid disease
       Acromegalic myopathy
       Steroid myopathy

4. *Genetically determined myopathies*
   (a) *Muscular dystrophies*
       Duchenne muscular dystrophy
       Becker muscular dystrophy
       Limb-girdle muscular dystrophy
       Facio-scapulo-humeral muscular dystrophy
       Scapulo-peroneal syndrome
       Oculo-pharyngeal muscular dystrophy
       Ocular myopathy

   (b) *Myotonic syndromes*
       Myotonic dystrophy
       Myotonia congenita
       Other myotonic syndromes

   (c) *Metabolic myopathies*
       Glycogenoses, e.g. McArdle's disease
       Disorders of lipid metabolism, e.g. carnitine deficiency
       Mitochondrial myopathies
       Periodic paralyses
       Malignant hyperpyrexia
       Myoglobinurias

(d) *Benign myopathies of childhood*
Central core and multicore disease
Myotubular myopathy
Nemaline myopathy
Congenital fibre-type disproportion
Congenital muscular dystrophy
Other rare syndromes

NEUROGENIC DISORDERS

1. *Disorders of anterior horn cells*
Spinal muscular atrophy (SMA)
Type 1 Werdnig–Hoffmann disease
Type 2 Intermediate SMA
Type 3 Juvenile onset Kugelberg–Welander disease
Type 4 Adult onset
Motor neuron disease
Poliomyelitis
Other anterior horn cell disorders

2. *Disorders of motor nerve roots*
Cervical and lumbar spondylosis with root compression
Malignant infiltration of nerve roots
Brachial neuritis (neuralgic amyotrophy)

3. *Peripheral neuropathies*
   (a) *Acquired polyneuropathies*
      (i) *metabolic*
         Diabetes mellitus
         Alcoholic neuropathy
         Renal and hepatic disease
         Vitamin deficiencies, e.g. B_{12} deficiency
      (ii) *Inflammatory polyradiculoneuropathy* (Guillain–Barré syndrome)
      (iii) *Drug-induced and toxic neuropathies*
         e.g. tri-ortho-cresyl phosphate poisoning, isoniazid neuropathy
      (iv) *Associated with malignant disease*
      (v) *Infections*, e.g. leprosy, diphtheria
      (vi) *Associated with collagen vascular disease*
         e.g. polyartertis nodosa and other vasculitides, rheumatoid arthritis

   (b) *Acquired mononeuropathies*
   Entrapment and compressive, e.g. carpal tunnel syndrome
   Traumatic
   Mononeuritis multiplex

   (c) *Genetically determined polyneuropathies*
   Charcot–Marie–Tooth syndrome
   Hereditary sensory neuropathies
   Amyloid neuropathy
   Porphyric neuropathy
   Metachromatic leukodystrophy
   Other rare syndromes, e.g. Refsum's disease

4. *Disorders of Neuromuscular transmission* (end plate disorders)
    Myasthenia gravis
    Myasthenic syndromes

1.4   Clinical features of neuromuscular disease

In the majority of patients in whom muscle biopsy is performed, the major problem is *weakness*. In most primary disorders of muscle, i.e. the myopathies, weakness is predominantly proximal, affecting the pelvic girdle muscles more severely than the shoulder girdle muscles. Proximal weakness is also a feature of spinal muscular atrophy, a disorder in which muscular weakness and atrophy develops as a result of progressive loss of anterior horn cells. In some peripheral neuropathies in which there is involvement of spinal roots as well of the peripheral nerves, e.g. Guillain-Barré polyradiculoneuropathy, proximal weakness may also occur but, in general, peripheral neuropathies are characterized by distal weakness, which is usually symmetrical, and distal sensory loss or paraesthesiae. In peripheral neuropathies the tendon reflexes are often absent, particularly the ankle and finger jerks and, if present, atrophy is also characteristically distal. In myopathies the tendon reflexes are usually present, although in Duchenne dystrophy, and in myotonic dystrophy, they are often reduced.

In most inherited myopathies and dystrophies, *proximal weakness* is symmetrical, but particular muscle groups are often selectively involved. For example, in Duchenne dystrophy, weakness of the hip flexors and extensors, quadriceps and tibialis anterior is often prominent. In limb–girdle muscular dystrophy the biceps and periscapular muscles are particularly weak and in facio-scapulo-humeral muscular dystrophy, facial, triceps, biceps and periscapular muscles are mainly affected. Other rare variants, such as scapulo-peroneal atrophy and quadriceps myopathy, are recognized. In myotonic dystrophy facial and distal limb weakness, also involving small hand muscles, is characteristic, and there is marked weakness and atrophy of neck flexor muscles.

Pseudohypertrophy, a clinical phenomenon in which weak muscles appear enlarged and unusually firm to palpation, is a particular feature of Duchenne dystrophy, in which it especially involves periscapular, deltoid and gastrocnemius muscles, but it also occurs in some patients with limb–girdle dystrophy and, rarely, in hypothyroid myopathy and certain other metabolic myopathies. Involvement of the bulbar musculature is characteristic of myasthenia gravis and motor neuron disease. It also occurs in myotonic dystrophy and in the rare disorder, oculo-pharyngeal dystrophy, but it is uncommon in other myopathies.

Muscular wasting is a feature of most progressive myopathies, and usually occurs in the distribution of the weakness. However, wasting is also a feature of neurogenic disorders. In the latter wasting may be accompanied by spontaneous fasciculation. This is an important and diagnostic feature of motor neuron disease, but it also occurs in some patients with spinal root lesions and, rarely, in thyrotoxicosis. In spinal muscular atrophies spontaneous fasciculation is uncommon, but fasciculation may occur after exercise and coarse tremulous contraction of individual muscle bundles can be recognized. In Werdnig–Hoffmann disease (infantile spinal muscular atrophy), however, fasciculation occurs at rest, especially in the tongue.

Myotonia consists of persistent contraction of a muscle or of part of a muscle after cessation of voluntary contraction. It can be recognized by its electromyographic features. It is usually a familial disturbance and may occur as an isolated clinical finding (e.g. myotonia congenita) or in association with other features of neuromuscular disease as in myotonic dystrophy or periodic paralysis.

Fatiguability is a common symptom noted not only by patients with neuromuscular diseases, but by patients with depression and as a reaction to undue psychological stress. It is thus difficult to define unless it is accompanied by definite evidence of a decrease in effort tolerance, or by the development of objective muscular weakness during exertion or movement. Fatiguability is particularly associated with myasthenia gravis. In this disorder weakness can usually be demonstrated by clinical tests of individual muscles during tonic or repeated movement. Commonly used tests include fist-clenching, abduction of the shoulder, and prolonged upward gaze leading to ptosis, but bulbar weakness is often evident during prolonged conversation or chewing. Fatiguability is also a feature of motor neuron disease, and of certain metabolic myopathies, particularly the mitochondrial myopathies. In polymyositis fatiguability is also a common complaint, especially in the early stages.

Muscular pain and stiffness occurs in inflammatory myopathies, in which it is particularly prominent in the mornings, or after rest, and may be particularly relieved by exercise. Similar symptoms occur in patients with inflammatory joint disease and it may be difficult for the clinician to be certain whether or not there is muscular involvement in such cases. Muscular pain is a particularly prominent feature of polymyalgia rheumatica, although weakness is usually only slight in this condition. Muscular pain also occurs in certain metabolic myopathies, especially myxoedema and McArdle's syndrome of myophosphorylase deficiency. In these patients muscular pain, stiffness or cramp usually develops during exercise, although it may be relieved with continued exercise. In neurogenic disorders, including peripheral neuropathies, muscular pain is unusual. However, cramps at rest and with exercise are common in motor neuron disease, and severe muscular pain and tenderness may occur in Guillain-Barré syndrome and in alcoholic neuropathy.

Many neuromuscular diseases are accompanied by features of *involvement of other organs*. For example, in inflammatory myopathies there may be skin or joint involvement, in myotonic dystrophy cataract, diabetes mellitus and other features may coexist, in Duchenne dystrophy cardiac involvement is common, and in certain hereditary neuropathies pes cavus and other skeletal deformities are often found. These additional features may lead to recognition of the hereditary nature of the disorder. Careful enquiry about a possible family history is always important in the diagnosis of neuromuscular disorders.

The *age of onset* of symptoms is also important in diagnosis. In general, most hereditary conditions have specific patterns of presentation and progression and these can be readily recognized by experienced clinicians.

1.5 Methods of investigation

A wide variety of different tests can be used to assess patients with neuromuscular disorders but most of these are applicable only in rare instances. For example; the ischaemic lactate test is used in the diagnosis of McArdle's myophosphorylase deficiency. A low blood potassium level, often induced by exercise or by a glucose load, is important in the diagnosis of hypokalaemic periodic paralysis; various quantitative biochemical assays are used in the diagnosis of metabolic myopathies; thyroid function tests are useful in thyrotoxic and hypothyroid myopathies. Tests for myoglobinuria may be helpful on some occasions; and measurement of serum immunoglobulins can be used in the diagnosis of some inflammatory myopathies, paraprotein-associated neuropathies, and polyarteritis. However, the most useful laboratory test is the measurement of 'muscle enzyme' levels in the blood.

Although a number of different enzymes may be released from muscle in neuromuscular diseases, only aldolase, pyruvate kinase and creatine kinase (CK) levels are useful in diagnosis. In most laboratories CK levels are preferred, since they provide a more sensitive indication of active muscular disease. The CK level is raised when muscle breakdown occurs, or when the muscle fibre membranes are abnormal, as in Duchenne dystrophy, allowing the muscle CK_{MM} isoenzyme to leak from the muscle cells into the circulation. In most laboratories CK isoenzyme assays are not available and the total venous blood CK level is measured. It is sometimes important to recognize that CK levels are affected by exercise and by the phase of the menstrual cycle, particularly if CK levels are being used in young women for genetic counselling when there is a risk of the carrier state for Duchenne dystrophy.

Since the CK level varies with the extent of muscle fibre damage, and with the muscle bulk, the level tends to be highest in the early and most active stages of a disease, and to be lowest at the end-stage, when there is marked muscle atrophy. The CK level is also relatively low during healing stages of inflammatory myopathies, and it may fall during steroid therapy, even if the disease remains active. In metabolic myopathies the CK level is usually normal since muscle destruction is not a feature of these disorders; if muscle fibre necrosis occurs, as in McArdle's disease, the CK level may be transiently raised. In neurogenic disorders the CK level is usually normal, but it may be slightly raised in chronic neurogenic disorders.

In the past, 24-hour urinary creatine/creatinine ratios were used for the diagnosis of progressive muscular disorders as an index of muscle bulk and muscle cell necrosis, but they are now little used. Recently, the 24-hour urinary 3-methylhistidine excretion has been used as a measure of muscle catabolism.

Electrocardiography is an important investigation since it provides evidence of an associated cardiomyopathy, e.g. in Duchenne dystrophy and Friedreich's ataxia.

Electromyography (EMG) is much used in the diagnosis of myopathic and neurogenic disorders. The technique consists both of needle electrode sampling of electrical activity in muscles at rest and during slight, graded muscular contraction, and of measurement of motor and sensory nerve conduction velocities. In the investigation of proximal weakness, the commonest presenting feature of patients submitted to muscle biopsy, needle EMG is particularly useful. Spontaneous electrical activity in resting muscle is uncommon except in neurogenic disorders, in which *fibrillations* representing spontaneous contractions of denervated muscle fibres, and *fasciculations*, representing spontaneous firing of parts or all of a motor unit, may occur. Fibrillations also occur rarely in myopathic disorders, in which segmental muscle necrosis may cause denervation of part of a muscle fibre by separating it from its nerve supply. Myotonic discharges can also be recognized during electrode insertion or movement.

During voluntary activation of a muscle the electrophysiological features of individual motor unit action potentials can be recognized, and the pattern and extent of their recruitment during increased activation can be studied. In neurogenic disorders individual potentials are larger and more complex than normal, owing to enlargement of the motor unit by reinnervation from axonal sprouts derived from surviving motor units. In myopathic disorders, however, individual potentials are smaller than normal, and usually shorter in duration, although they may also show increased complexity. This is due to loss of individual muscle fibres within the motor unit and to changes in muscle fibre size. The latter causes increased variability in the speed of propagation of the action potential in individual fibres.

In myasthenia gravis, the abnormality of neuromuscular transmission at the motor end-plates results in fatiguability, which can be studied electrophysiologically. The size of the muscle action potential during repetitive stimulation of its nerve is progressively reduced in most myasthenic patients. This diagnosis can also be made by assay of circulating acetylcholine receptor antibodies.

Nerve conduction studies are especially useful in the diagnosis of peripheral neuropathies, and may help differentiate predominantly axonal from demyelinating neuropathies. They are particularly used in the diagnosis and management of entrapment neuropathies. Nerve conduction studies are usually normal in anterior horn cell disorders.

1.6 Indications for muscle biopsy

Most muscle biopsies are usually arranged by rheumatologists, physicians, neurologists, or paediatricians. Rheumatologists and physicians are concerned particularly with patients with inflammatory muscle disease, usually associated with autoimmune disorders; neurologists use muscle biopsies for a wide variety of neuromuscular disorders and paediatricians are involved with a different group of disorders, especially 'floppy baby' syndromes, muscular dystrophy and childhood-type dermatomyositis.

The main indications for muscle biopsy are shown in Table 1.2. Of these the most common are in the diagnosis of inflammatory muscle disease and in the diagnosis of proximal weakness of unknown cause. In relation to the frequency of muscle biopsy for these indications, biopsies in infants and children are rare except in specialized centres, since the childhood myopathies and dystrophies are themselves uncommon disorders. In general, muscle biopsies in patients with suspected autoimmune vasculitis are unlikely to provide useful information unless the muscle biopsied is clinically involved, either by tenderness or by weakness.

1.7 Selection of muscle for biopsy

Most biopsies are taken from the deltoid, biceps brachii or quadriceps femoris muscles but triceps and gastrocnemius muscles are sometimes chosen if these muscles are considered more likely to show abnormality.

Table 1.2 Indications for muscle biopsy

---

1. Inflammatory muscle disease before beginning treatment.
2. Proximal weakness of uncertain cause whether myopathic or neurogenic in adults and children, including 'floppy baby' syndromes.
3. Hereditary myopathies and muscular dystrophies.
4. To exclude treatable disorder, e.g. polymyositis, in patients in whom motor neuron disease is suspected.
5. Suspected metabolic myopathies, particularly in patients with muscle cramps, stiffness or tenderness.
6. Autoimmune vasculitis, especially polyarteritis nodosa, even in the absence of muscular symptoms.
7. Other systemic disorders, e.g. sarcoidosis, infestations.
8. To assess the effects of steroid treatment in the management of polymyositis, particularly in relation to the development of steroid myopathy.
9. Occasionally in carrier detection in female siblings or other close female relatives of boys with Duchenne dystrophy.
10. Diagnosis of malignant hyperpyrexia syndrome by *in vitro* test.
11. Research; e.g. exercise physiology, pathological and immunological studies, etc.

Generally deltoid, biceps brachii and quadriceps femoris muscles are preferred for biopsy because no disability is likely to result from the biopsy. In addition, skin sutures are not under tension, the biopsy can be easily orientated for precise transverse and longitudinal sections, and the normal features of these muscles are well understood. The biceps brachii is particularly suitable because it contains approximately equal numbers of the different histochemical types of muscle fibre. In both deltoid and quadriceps femoris muscles there are variations in fibre type proportions in different parts of the muscle.

Muscles previously used for EMG should not be used for muscle biopsy because artefact caused by the needle electrode may lead to difficulty in interpretation. Indeed, marked abnormalities (needle myopathy) have been described (Engel, 1967). It is important to biopsy a muscle which is clinically affected, but muscles showing marked wasting should be avoided, since only end-stage fibrosis and fat replacement may be found. In neurogenic disorders moderately weak muscles should be biopsied whenever possible, but in myopathic conditions less severely involved muscles often show characteristic abnormalities and the choice of muscle is thus less important. In inflammatory muscle disease tender muscles are particularly likely to yield diagnostic information.

The development of needle muscle biopsy, a technique largely restricted to the lateral part of the quadriceps muscle, has encouraged clinicians to consider muscle biopsy in patients in whom open muscle biopsy would not be undertaken, and has allowed repeat biopsy to be undertaken when necessary. Further, it can sometimes be used in conjunction with open biopsy of an arm muscle to compare the distribution of abnormality in the upper and lower limbs.

References

Brandstater, M. E. and Lambert, E. H. (1973), Motor unit anatomy. In *New Developments in Electromyography and Clinical Neurophysiology*, Vol. 1 (ed. J. E. Desmedt), Karger, Basel, pp. 14–22.

Dubowitz, V. and Pearse, A. G. E. (1960), Reciprocal relationship of phosphorylase and oxidative enzymes in skeletal muscle. *Nature*, **185**, 701.

Edstrom, L. and Kugelberg, E. (1968), Histochemical composition, distribution of fibres and fatiguability of single motor units. *J. Neurol. Neurosurg. Psychiatry*, **31**, 424–33.

Engel, W. K. (1967), Focal myopathic changes produced by electromyographic and hypodermic needles. *Arch. Neurol.*, **16**, 509–13.

Swash, M. and Schwartz, M. S. (1981), *Neuromuscular Diseases: A Practical Approach to Diagnosis*, Springer-Verlag, Berlin, Heidelberg and New York.

Walton, J. N. and Gardner-Medwin, D. (1981), Classification of neuromuscular disease In *Disorders of Voluntary Muscle*, 4th edn (ed. J. N. Walton), Churchill-Livingstone, Edinburgh.

2   Laboratory methods

There are two techniques available for muscle biopsy. *Open biopsy* is carried out by a surgeon in the operating theatre, usually under local anaesthesia, but *needle biopsy* (Fig. 2.1) can be performed at any convenient location (Edwards, 1971). In order to obtain a specimen free of artefact and thus suitable both for light and electron microscopy it is important to maintain a scrupulous technique in handling the biopsy. In the case of open muscle biopsy the surgeon and his assistants must be aware that clamping, stretching, squeezing or drying the muscle tissue will all lead to unacceptable artefacts which may well interfere with proper interpretation of the biopsy. Muscle obtained by open biopsy should therefore be delivered to the waiting technician in the operating theatre so that the specimen can be dealt with immediately. Needle biopsy carries with it the advantage that the biopsy specimen is protected within the needle and is not therefore likely to be handled before it is given to the technician. Another source of artefact is the injection of local anaesthetic deeply into the muscle at the biopsy site. This results in disruption of the muscle tissue. Local anaesthetic should therefore only be injected into the skin and subcutaneous tissue. Since the perimysium contains pain fibres the incision or needle thrust into the muscle will, inevitably, be slightly painful, but this is a penalty that should be accepted in order to obtain high quality histological preparations.

2.1   Preparation of the biopsy

Fixation in formol-saline, with subsequent paraffin-embedding, is of limited value in muscle pathology since it does not allow the use of enzyme histochemical or ultrastructural techniques. Its place is restricted to autopsy studies and as a means of conveniently storing material which can be used for study by conventional histological staining techniques. Thus stains for fibrous tissue, trichrome stains, and methods for calcium, RNA, DNA and glycogen, can be utilized. In addition, immunoperoxidase

14

Fig. 2.1 (a) and (b) The modified Bergström needle (UCH needle) used for muscle biopsy to show the hollow cavity into which the biopsy is taken.

reactions can also be applied. However, modern muscle histopathology depends primarily on a series of standardized enzyme histochemical reactions, applied to unfixed frozen tissue: without these, the diagnostic potential of the muscle biopsy is greatly restricted. In addition, most of the classical histological techniques can be adapted for use in frozen tissue, and most modern enzyme histochemical reactions produce permanent results, so that the slides can be stored for future comparative study. Electron microscopy is applicable in certain diagnostic situations and it is useful to fix part of the biopsy for possible future study with the electron microscope, even if this material is not always processed fully.

The first step in preparation of the muscle biopsy is thus to select tissue for ultrastructural studies. Tiny cubes of tissue, no larger than 1 mm in any dimension, are cut from the biopsied muscle tissue and fixed for up to 4 h in cooled glutaraldelyde or Karnovsky fixative. Routine plastic-embedding methods may then be followed, or the tissue may be stored for some time in buffer before embedding is carried out. It is important not to delay fixation of tissue for electron microscopy for more than a few minutes, in order to avoid swelling and disruption of mitochondria, and of the sarcoplasmic tubular system. In general, the smaller the tissue blocks taken into fixative, the better will be the results. It is usually quite easy to make sure that the blocks are cut at right angles to the orientation of the muscle fibres, so that true transverse and longitudinal sections can be prepared after embedding.

The remainder of the biopsy is snap-frozen for light microscopy. The materials needed for snap-freezing muscle are listed in Table 2.1. Isopentane is cooled in a small metal container suspended in the mouth of a thermos flask of liquid nitrogen. Isopentane solidifies at this temperature ($-160°C$) and it is necessary to remove the isopentane container from the flask when the first solid-phase isopentane appears. The biopsy, moistened if necessary with buffered saline, or Ringer's solution, is cut cleanly with a sharp scalpel blade into small pieces no larger than 4 mm × 2 mm. The longer side of the specimen should be orientated longitudinally with the muscle fibres. Great care must be taken not to transfix the muscle specimen with a needle, or crush it with forceps or scissors since this produces marked artefact.

Table 2.1 Equipment used for snap-freezing muscle biopsies in the operating theatre, ward or outpatients department

---

Small open-topped thermos flask half filled with liquid nitrogen
Bottle of isopentane
Small metal drug container, suspended with stiff wire in the mouth of the flask
Long and short forceps
Scissors
Sharp, new, scalpel blades
Small cork discs (diameter 0.5 cm or less; thickness < 1 mm)
Tissue-Tek(R)
Small plastic containers suitable for storage of muscle specimens in liquid nitrogen or $-70°C$ refrigerator
Swabs
Ringer's solution
EM fixative (pre-cooled to 4°C)
A few hypodermic needles (used for removing tissue from shaft of muscle biopsy needle)
A pair of asbestos gloves
Form for clinical details, etc
Labels and pencil

Each piece of muscle tissue is mounted on a separate tiny, thin cork disc, previously prepared, using a small blob of Tissue-Tek(R) or other adhesive, and the cork disc and muscle tissue is then dropped lightly into the cooled isopentane. It is thus snap-frozen. It is usually possible to orientate the muscle tissue so that its fibres are arranged longitudinally or vertically on the cork disc. Transverse sections are more useful than longitudinal sections in diagnostic work, so most blocks should be arranged with the muscle fibres in the vertical plane. Occasionally, especially in biopsies taken from bipennate muscles, orientation is difficult and the muscle biopsy should then be taken, moistened with Ringer's solution, to a dissection stereomicroscope for proper orientation.

The frozen biopsy with its attached cork disc (Fig. 2.2) should be removed from the isopentane after a minute or so, placed into a previously cooled small plastic container (itself brought to the biopsy in liquid nitrogen) and then carried back to the laboratory immersed in the flask of liquid nitrogen itself. The specimen may then be stored in a refrigerator kept at −70°C or in liquid nitrogen, in a special container. Specimens can be preserved indefinitely in liquid nitrogen without losing their enzyme reactivity and without fear of loss of material from mechanical or electrical failure in a refrigerator. It is thus not necessary to process part of a biopsy into paraffin, after formalin fixation, for permanent storage. Furthermore, a small specimen is also available embedded in resin in the EM laboratory.

In some laboratories a freezing mixture of methanol and dry ice is used for cooling isopentane to an appropriate temperature for snap-freezing tissue. This method works well, although the freezing mixture is not at such a low temperature as when the liquid nitrogen method is used. This freezing mixture is cumbersome and so not easy to transport to the ward or operating theatre; we therefore prefer to use liquid nitrogen. It is possible to snap-freeze muscle biopsies directly in the flask of liquid nitrogen, by first coating the biopsy in talc before immersing it in the liquid nitrogen. The layer of talc helps to exclude air bubbles from the surface of the biopsy, thus facilitating rapid and uniform cooling of the muscle tissue. Failure to use talc means that a layer of air 'boils off' from the surface of the biopsy. This irregular heat flux from the biopsy causes artefact in the tissue, both from ice crystal formation within muscle fibres, and from cracking of the tissue. Finally, it is best to avoid trying to quench large muscle biopsies pinned to small matchsticks, or held in double Spencer Wells clamps because these methods involve cooling large volumes of material of varying thermal conductivity and this frequently results in unacceptable ice crystal artefact.

Fig. 2.2   Muscle biopsy specimen on cork disc, ready for sectioning. The cork layer, surrounded by ice, is frozen onto the precooled metal chuck.

2.2   Cutting sections

Sections of snap-frozen tissue are cut in a cryostat, at a temperature of about −20°C. Since the tissue is stored in liquid nitrogen at −160°C there is a marked temperature difference between the tissue and cryostat temperatures. The tissue block is fixed to a cooled chuck by a drop of water, which freezes the cork disc to the chuck; the cork insulates the biopsy itself from the relatively warm chuck, but the latter may itself be cooled to −160°C in liquid nitrogen and this manoeuvre helps to prevent ice crystals forming in the tissue. When the chuck has been fixed in the cryostat a little time should be allowed to elapse before sections are cut with a cooled knife.

A series of 6 to 12 transverse sections, each 5–8 μm thick should be cut. It is sometimes useful to cut a similar series of longitudinal sections but most of the relevant information required for diagnosis can be obtained from transverse sections. A larger series of transverse sections may be required, particularly when the longitudinal extent of a particular abnormality is of importance. When the sections have been cut the cork disc and biopsy can be removed from the chuck by a sharp blow with a knife on the layer of ice between them, and the specimen can be returned to the liquid nitrogen tissue-storage container or refrigerator (−70°C) until it is required again.

2.3 Histological methods

A standard series of histological and enzyme histochemical methods (Fig. 2.3) should be carried out on each biopsy (Table 2.2). This series is intended to provide a basis for histopathological appraisal of the biopsy, to allow study of the distribution of different fibre types, and to identify a range of normal and abnormal structures within muscle fibres.

2.3.1 Haematoxylin and eosin (HE)

This well-known histological stain is the most useful of all the techniques used in muscle biopsy work. In cryostat sections the muscle fibres are free of fixation artefact and thus appear as slightly rounded structures, neatly interdigitating with each other and with their endomysial capillaries (Fig. 2.3). Abnormal variation in fibre size, fibres which have lost their normal granularity, basophilic regenerating fibres, necrotic fibres and small pyknotic fibres can all easily be recognized. Any inflammatory cell response can be identified, in relation to muscle fibres, interstitial tissue or blood vessels. Nerve fibres can also be studied within muscle biopsies in HE stains. Rare abnormalities, such as granulomas, parasites or tumour deposits are also best seen in the HE preparation. However, fat cells and fibrous tissue are not well delineated.

2.3.2 Reduced nicotine adenine dinucleotide tetrazolium reductase (NADH)

This oxidative enzyme reaction identifies mitochondria which contain the cell's oxidative enzymes, but there is also a less specific reaction with sarcoplasmic tubules. Since both mitochondria and sarcoplasmic tubules are located between the myofibrils this enzyme reaction delineates the intermyofibrillar anatomy of the muscle fibres. The reaction product is

Fig. 2.3 Normal muscle in serial transverse section (Needle biopsy), × 140. (a) PAS. The polygonal muscle fibres are interdigitated, and the endomysial nuclei are subsarcolemmal. The different fibre types usually cannot be differentiated reliably in this technique; the fibres with the more marked glycogen content are Type 1 fibres. (b) ATPase, pH 9.4. In the alkali-stable ATPase reaction Type 2 fibres react darkly and Type 1 fibres appear pale. Note the Type 1 fibre surrounded by dark Type 2 fibres to the left of the centre of the illustration.

(c) ATPase, pH 4.3. This reaction is the converse of the result at pH 9.4. The pale fibre noted in (b) now reacts darkly, and its surrounding fibres are pale. (d) NADH. In this technique the granular intermyofibrillar material, including mitochondria, reacts darkly. Type 1 fibres, rich in mitochondria, appear dark, but fibres of both types react to some extent. The Type 2 fibres often show varying degrees of reactivity, but the subtypes cannot be consistently identified in this technique.

Table 2.2 Routine series of histological methods for muscle biopsies

Haematoxylin and eosin (HE)
Nicotine adenine dinucleotide dehydrogenase tetrazolium reductase (NADH)
Myosin adenosine triphosphatase (ATPase) – preincubated at pH 9.4, 4.6 and 4.3, respectively
Modified Gomori trichrome
Periodic acid Schiff (PAS)
Oil red O/Ehrlich's haematoxylin
Verhoeff van Gieson

seen as a coarsely granular or reticulate deposition throughout the fibre, except in zones occupied by subsarcolemmal nuclei. Two fibre types can be recognized by the density of the reaction but in most muscles a large number of fibres with an intermediate reaction occur (Fig. 2.3). Fibres with a strong reaction represent fibres dependent on oxidative metabolism, the slow-twitch Type 1 fibres. Less strongly reactive fibres are capable of anaerobic, glycolytic metabolism; these are the fast-twitch Type 2 fibres (Table 2.3). Sections prepared for NADH tend to lift off glass slides, thus making microscopy at higher magnifications difficult. This can be prevented by partially fixing the dried section on the slide with 70% alcohol before starting the enzyme reaction.

Succinic dehydrogenase (SDH) may also be identified by an enzyme histochemical technique. This reaction is specific for SDH and thus for mitochondria, a useful point when a mitochondrial myopathy is suspected.

2.3.2   Myosin ATPase methods

Fibre typing is usually carried out, by convention, on myosin ATPase preparations (Table 2.3). The currently used classification of fibre types in man was devised in myosin ATPase preparations preincubated at pH 9.4, 4.6 and 4.3 (Brooke and Kaiser, 1970). Other classifications of fibre types, based on different histochemical techniques, have been devised but these are complex and of little practical value (Romanul, 1964). With preincubation at pH 9.4 two fibre types can be differentiated, darkly reacting Type 2 fibres and lightly reacting Type 1 fibres. This reaction is reversed in the preincubation at pH 4.3. In intermediate preincubations, usually carried out at pH 4.6, three fibre types can be recognized, consisting of Type 1, Type 2A and Type 2B fibres (Table 2.3). At this pH, Type 1 and Type 2B fibres are both dark; the Type 1 fibres are usually darker than the Type 2B fibres (Fig. 2.3). In the myosin ATPase reaction, myofibrils react positively; this reaction thus demonstrates the myofibril-

Table 2.3 Classification of muscle fibre types in standard histological methods (from Swash and Schwartz, 1981)

	Type 1	Type 2A	Type 2B
Myosin ATPase			
pH 9.4	Pale	Dark	Dark
pH 4.6	Dark	Pale	Intermediate
pH 4.3	Dark	Pale	Pale
NADH	Dark	Intermediate	Intermediate
PAS	Pale	Dark	Intermediate
Oil red O			
(lipid droplets)	Plentiful	Sparse	Sparse
Myophosphorylase	Pale	Dark	Dark
HE	Darker red	Red	Red
Physiological characteristics	Slow twitch	Fast twitch: Fatigue-resistant	Fast twitch: Rapidly fatiguing

lar material itself. The distribution and packing density of myofibrils may thus be assessed by this method.

2.3.4 Periodic acid Schiff method (PAS)

This technique is used to demonstrate glycogen, and membranous structures containing mucopolysaccharide, glycoproteins, mucoprotein, glycolipids and phospholipids (Fig. 2.3). The presence of glycogen can be established by incubating a second section after predigestion with diastase; any remaining reaction product must then be due to cellular or tubular membranes. The PAS method does not produce a reaction which can easily be quantified, but generally two fibre types can be recognized (Table 2.3) and any increase in the glycogen content of muscle fibres can be established. The technique is best carried out after alcohol prefixation of the dried section, which prevents washing-out of glycogen during the preparative procedure. The method may also be combined with a haematoxylin or other nuclear counterstain, which aids identification of individual fibres in the serial sections.

2.3.6 Modified Gomori trichrome

This trichrome method, modified for use in cryostat sections, has become deservedly popular in muscle biopsies. Muscle fibres stain greenish-blue, the intermyofibrillar tubules, mitochondria and membrane-bound fat droplets appear a bright red and the endomysial connective/fibrous tissue stains green. Nuclei appear reddish-brown and are thus easily seen. The popularity of this stain derives from the ease with which necrotic or hyaline fibres can be seen, and abnormal intrasarcoplasmic inclusions, such as rod bodies, and abnormalities of mitochondria or of the sarcoplasmic tubular system can also be recognized. The presence of these abnormalities can be confirmed by electron microscopy.

In well-prepared Gomori-stained sections two fibre types can be recognized by their differential sarcoplasmic staining, just as in well-stained HE preparations. The method depends very much on good histological techniques; dried sections, too thick sections, or stale Gomori stain will all lead to poor results, often with areas of blotchy pink pigment across the section.

2.3.6   Oil red O/Ehrlich's haematoxylin

Neutral lipids can be demonstrated by several methods including oil red O and Sudan black. The oil red O technique produces a bright red reaction which is easily seen as small red droplets in the fibres. The Type 1 fibres contain larger and more numerous lipid droplets than the Type 2 fibres. A haematoxylin counterstain is useful because not only does it indicate the position of the muscle fibre nuclei (Fig. 2.3), but it picks out basophilic regenerating fibres particularly clearly. In some myopathies lipid droplets accumulate, as in carnitine deficiency and in steroid myopathy.

2.3.7   Verhoejf van Gieson stain

Fibrous tissue appears red in this method and this is sometimes a useful technique for the assessment of increased interstitial fibrous tissue in myopathies. Similar delineation of fibrous tissue can be made with the Gomori method, but the Verhoeff van Gieson is easier to carry out satisfactorily. It may also be usefully combined with Hart's method for elastic tissue.

2.3.8   Other useful histological techniques

A number of other techniques are sometimes useful in diagnosis, particularly when specific problems arise. For example, the myophosphorylase technique, formerly used for muscle fibre typing, is useful when McArdle's disease (myophosphorylase deficiency) is suspected. It is often helpful to use specific histological methods for intrasarcoplasmic RNA and DNA. Methods are also available for intracellular calcium deposition and such as von Kossa's method and alizarin red. Immunoperoxidase methods for demonstration of serum immunoproteins in muscle fibres or in inflammatory cells, or of immune complexes in capillaries are occasionally of value. Some of these methods, suitable for cryostat sections, are listed in Table 2.4.

Table 2.4 Special histological techniques applicable to cryostat sections of muscle

Method	Indication
Toluidine blue	A quick method, comparable to HE as a screening stain. It may also be used to demonstrate metachromasia
Acid phosphatase	Demonstrates autophagic vacuoles in degenerating and many regenerating muscle fibres
Acridine orange	A fluorescence method specific for RNA
Methylgreen pyronin	Demonstrates RNA (red) and DNA (green). Increased sarcoplasmic RNA is an indication of protein synthesis, and thus muscle fibre regeneration. Increased sarcoplasmic DNA is found in degenerating or necrotic fibres
Myophosphorylase	(See Table 2.3). Prominent in Type 2 fibres. The enzyme is absent in McArdle's disease
Phosphofructokinase	Deficiency of this enzyme rarely occurs in a syndrome similar to McArdle's disease
Von Kossa or alizarin red	Calcium
Acetylcholinesterase with or without silver impregnation	Useful for demonstrating motor end-plates
Non-specific esterase	Increased in denervated fibres.
Immunoperoxidase methods	For immunoproteins. These methods are generally not useful in routine diagnosis

2.3.9 Plastic-embedded material

Semithin sections of plastic or resin-embedded muscle are of great value (Fig. 2.4). Indeed, in many instances, almost as much information may be gained from study of semithin sections as may be obtained from electron microscopy itself, especially if high magnifications or phase contrast

(a)

(b)

Fig. 2.4 (a) Drawing of the sliding filament structure of the myofilament in longitudinal and transverse planes. Compare with the ultrastructural appearance in the longitudinal ($\times$ 18 000) (b) and transverse ($\times$ 46 800) electron micrographs (c). (After Landon, 1982.)

microscopy are used. In most laboratories toluidine blue stains are used, but other methods are available. Inclusions within muscle fibres, or abnormalities of subcellular organelles such as tubules, or mitochondria, can often be recognized in these semithin sections.

2.3.10   Electron microscopy

Transmission electron microscopy was used to formulate modern concepts of the subcellular organization of muscle fibres, and the structure of the sliding filaments responsible for muscular contraction (Fig. 2.4). However, the advent of enzyme histochemistry and of toluidine blue staining of semithin sections has made electron microscopy less useful in routine diagnosis of muscle biopsies than might at first be supposed. The main value of ultrastructural studies by transmission electron microscopy is thus as a research technique. Generally, transmission electron microscopy cannot be expected to provide diagnostic information if no abnormality is discerned in light microscopy. Ultrastructural studies have proven to be most useful in the investigation of the congenital or benign myopathies of childhood, in which specific abnormalities of diagnostic value may occur.

Freeze-fracture electron microscopy has been used in research on membrane structure in the muscular dystrophies, especially in Duchenne muscular dystrophy, and scanning electron microscopy may have a similar application. Neither of these techniques has, as yet, revealed abnormalities sufficiently specific to be used in clinical diagnosis.

2.3.11   Autopsy methods

Muscle obtained at autopsy is generally suitable for study by most of the histological and enzyme histological methods discussed above, provided that specimens comparable in size to those obtained at muscle biopsy are prepared by snap-freezing in isopentane cooled with liquid nitrogen. Most muscle enzymes can be demonstrated in autopsy specimens even as long as 48 h after death, particularly if the cadaver has been kept adequately cooled in a refrigerator. It is particularly important to prepare muscle specimens with these techniques at autopsy in order to study the distribution of abnormality in neuromuscular diseases and this has, so far, been much neglected in muscle pathology. Many neuromuscular diseases are still defined only in terms of their muscle biopsy appearances. Autopsies of patients dying with neuromuscular diseases should not therefore be restricted to the examination of a few proximal muscles, for example biceps brachii and quadriceps femoris, using only formalin-fixed, paraffin-embedded material. Instead, a wide selection of bulbar, and of proximal and distal, upper and lower limb, muscles should be studied in cryostat sections. Normal material has been investigated by Polgar et al. (1973) and by Johnson et al. (1973), who studied 36 different muscles at autopsy. Cryostat sections have considerable advantages over paraffin sections. Not only may enzyme reactions be utilized but the morphology of individual fibres is more easily studied. Paraffin-sections of muscle, even at autopsy, are prone to be marred by artefact from shrinkage, cracking and even from imperfect fixation.

Attempts to examine autopsied muscle samples by electron microscopy, however, produce unsatisfactory results because of post-mortem autolysis.

2.4 Histological techniques for other structures found in muscle

Muscle biopsies often contain small nerve fibre bundles and, less commonly, other structures, such as motor end-plates, muscle spindles, Golgi tendon organs and Pacinian corpuscles may be present. These may not easily be identified at first, but it is important to recognize them as normal structures in sections of muscle.

2.4.1   Nerve fibre bundles

These can be recognized in HE preparation by the characteristic bluish-red colour of myelin (Fig. 2.5). Silver impregnations such as Schofield's technique for frozen sections or the Glees and Marsland method for paraffin-embedded tissue may be useful. Most nerve fibre bundles are found in interfascicular planes.

Fig. 2.5 × 140; HE. Several small bundles of nerve fibres can be seen between and within fasciculi.

2.4.2   Motor end-plates

Motor end-plates are not frequently found in muscle biopsies since most biopsies are taken away from the motor point. They are difficult to recognize in HE (Fig. 2.6) or van Gieson stains and are not visualized in the routine enzyme preparations, but the acetylcholinesterase method demonstrates the end-plate apparatus in sectioned material, and a modification of this technique, described by Pestronk and Drachman (1979) enables it to be combined with silver impregnation in frozen material. Another technique, used for studies of motor end-plates in man, uses supravital methylene blue, injected into the muscle at the time of the biopsy (Fig. 2.7). This method can produce impregnations not only of the terminal nerve tree and preterminal axonal sprouts of the motor end-plates, but also of intramuscular nerve fibres.

Fig. 2.6   × 350; HE. Enlargement of Fig. 2.5. A motor end-plate can just be recognized, with its sole-plate nuclei (arrows), innervated by axons from a nearby intramuscular nerve bundle.

At autopsy the acetylcholinesterase method may be used up to 48 h or so after death. Paraffin-embedded or frozen sections can be used for silver impregnations and block impregnations have also been utilized.

2.4.3   Other intramuscular organelles

Muscle spindles are sometimes found in muscle biopsies, particularly in open biopsies (Fig. 3.4). Special techniques are available for studying the

Fig. 2.7 Methylene blue preparation. Normal rat motor end-plate. Note the preterminal axonal branching and the subneural, presynaptic apparatus.

innervation of these complex sensory receptors (see Swash and Fox, 1972).

2.4.4   Other studies on muscle biopsies

A number of quantitative biochemical assays of muscle enzyme activity, for example in suspected glycogen storage disorders, have been used for diagnosis, and similar techniques have recently applied to patients with mitochondrial myopathies in order to define the underlying mitochondrial metabolic disorder (Morgan-Hughes, 1982).

2.4.5   Artefacts

A number of artefacts occur both in frozen and paraffin-embedded muscle. In frozen muscle the most common artefact is due to ice crystal formation, which produces a speckled pattern of small holes in the muscle fibres (Fig. 2.8). These usually have sharply defined, rather concave borders, with sharp corners, but they can be confused with lipid droplets. When severe they may mar interpretation of the biopsy. They may be avoided by scrupulous attention to snap-freezing technique and, especially by care during section cutting. They are particularly likely to occur if the knife blade or the slides are warmer than the temperature of the muscle tissue. If a block is affected by ice-crystal artefact, the sections

Fig. 2.8　× 380; HE. Ice-crystal artefact. This artefact is often found in only part of a section – it may then result from differential warming or cooling in different parts of the section, during section cutting, or when fixing the block to the chuck in the cryostat.

can sometimes be improved by allowing the block to melt to room temperature, and then refreezing it. However, this often results in slight swelling of the fibres, shown by a rounded appearance.

Knife-cutting artefacts, consisting of ridges of variable thickness in the section, are fairly common and are usually due to vibration in the cryostat. Blunt knives may cause a similar abnormality, or lead to tears in the section. Folded sections, especially at one edge, usually result from poor technique during the enzyme or staining reactions. If a block is allowed to dry before snap-freezing, the fibres at its edge become shrunken, vitreous and excessively eosinophilic, an appearance which may easily be confused with the hypercontracted, hyalinised fibres found in Duchenne muscular dystrophy. Haemorrhage, displacing fibres in a fascicle, is invariably due to surgical trauma. Similarly, apparent oedematous displacement of fibres from each other in a fascicle may be due to local anaesthetic inadvertently injected into the muscle at the biopsy site.

Muscle biopsies prepared for paraffin sections are vulnerable to fixation artefact, in which muscle fibres undergo abrupt hypercontraction with loss of cross striations and loss of orientation. This can be avoided by pre-preparation in Ringer's solution for 15–30 min before fixation in buffered formol saline. Formalin-fixation of biopsied or autopsied muscle is best accomplished by pinning short narrow strips of muscle on to a card, in a slightly stretched state. Fixation should not be prolonged longer than a few hours or overnight if the best histological results are to be obtained. Paraffin-embedding should be carried out using a slow embedding schedule.

Muscle prepared for electron microscopy is also vulnerable to artefact (Mair and Tomé, 1972). Fixation should be accomplished as rapidly as possible after removal of tissue from the patient in order to avoid mitochondrial swelling. It should not be prolonged longer than about 4 hs, the muscle then being best stored in buffered saline prior to plastic-embedding.

References

Brooke, M. H. and Kaiser, K. K. (1970), Muscle fibre types: how many and what kind? *Arch. Neurol.*, **23**, 369–79.

Edwards, R. H. T. (1971), Percutaneous needle-biopsy of skeletal muscle in diagnosis and research. *Lancet*, **ii**, 593–6.

Johnson, M. A., Polgar, J., Weightman, D., Appleton, D. (1973), Data on the distribution of fibre types in thirty-six human muscles: an autopsy study. *J. Neurol. Sci.*, **18**, 111–29.

Landon, D. N. (1982), Skeletal muscle: normal morphology, development and innervation. In *Skeletal Muscle Pathology* (eds F. L. Mastaglia and J. N. Walton), Churchill Livingstone, Edinburgh, ch. 1, p. 187.

Mair, W. G. P. and Tomé, F. M. S. (1972), *Atlas of the Ultrastructure of Diseased Human Muscle*, Churchill Livingstone, Edinburgh.

Morgan-Hughes, J. A. (1982), Defects of the energy pathways of skeletal muscle. In *Recent Advances in Clinical neurology*, Vol. 3 (eds W. B. Matthews and G. H. Glaser), Churchill Livingstone, Edinburgh, pp. 1–46.

Pestronk, A. and Drachman, D. B. (1979), A new stain for quantitative measurement of sprouting at neuromuscular junctions. *Muscle Nerve* 1, 70–4.

Polgar, J., Johnson, M. A., Weightman, D., and Appleton, D. (1973), Data on fibre size in thirty-six human muscles: an autopsy study. *J. Neurol. Sci.*, **19**, 307–18.

Romanul, F. C. (1964), Enzymes in muscle. I. Histochemical studies of enzymes in individual muscle fibres. *Arch. Neurol.*, **11**, 355–8.

Swash, M. and Fox, K. P. (1972), Techniques for the demonstration of human muscle spindle innervation in neuromuscular disease. *J. Neurol. Sci*, **15**, 291–302.

Swash, M. and Schwartz, M. S. (1981), *Neuromuscular Diseases: A Practical Approach to Diagnosis and Management*, Springer-Verlag, Berlin, Heidelberg, New York.

3 Histological and morphometric characteristics of normal muscle

Muscle fibres in frozen sections, prepared as discussed in Chapter 2, normally take the form of irregular polygons with slightly rounded sides, in close apposition to each other. In an idealized cross section of normal muscle, if all muscle fibres were of equal size each fibre would conform to a hexagonal shape (Fig. 3.1), but Type 1, Type 2A and Type 2B fibres differ somewhat in their mean diameter and so there is variation not only in size, but in shape. In addition to the histological appearance of muscle fibres and of the endomysial and interfascicular tissue and organelles, the size of fibres, the distribution of fibres of different histochemical types and the relative predominance of different fibre types can be studied.

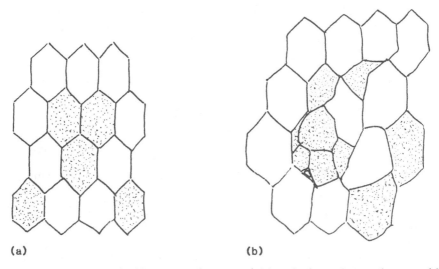

(a)   (b)

Fig. 3.1 If all muscle fibres were hexagonal (a) and of equal size, they would interdigitate in a regular pattern, but not all fibres conform to this shape. Fibres smaller than normal, or fibres with fewer 'sides' alter the pattern of interdigitation (b).

34

3.1   Fibre size

Muscle fibre size has usually been expressed as the lesser transverse diameter (Brooke and Engel, 1969), since this measurement is least affected by variations in the plane of section of the muscle fibre away from the true transverse plane. Fibre diameters can be measured simply with an eye piece micrometer calibrated against a graduated scale, or from photographic enlargements of transverse sections of muscle. Care must be taken either to measure *all* the fibres in a biopsy, however large or small, or to measure *all* the fibres contained within an arbitrary number, not less than 5, of different microscope fields, selected randomly in the biopsy. At least 100 fibres of each type should be measured. Sufficient fibres are usually available in needle muscle biopsies for these quantitative studies.

Fibre size increases with maturation (Fig. 3.2). At one year of age the mean fibre diameter is 16 μm and at age 10 years, 40 μm. It increases by 2 μm for each year to age 5 years and then by 3 μm for each year to age 9 years. Adult diameters are achieved between age 12 and 15 years (Table 3.1). In adult men most muscle fibres are within the range 40–80 μm diameter, and in adult women 30–70 μm. Fibres smaller than 20 μm, or larger than 100 μm diameter are not usually found in muscle. In childhood, Type 1 and Type 2 fibres are of similar size to each other. In adult women Type 1 fibres are larger than Type 2 fibres, but in men the reverse obtains. In normal subjects muscle fibre diameters have been thoroughly studied in the biceps brachii, lateral quadriceps and deltoid muscles (Table 3.1). Polgar *et al.* (1973) measured the mean diameters of Type 1 and Type 2 fibres in an autopsy study of 36 different human muscles in six male subjects. This study showed that Type 2 fibres were of larger diameter than Type 1 fibres in 90% of the muscles examined, but that this difference in mean diameter was usually not statistically significant. Both fibre types were equally variable in fibre size, with moderately large ranges of diameter values in individual subjects. In some muscles, the muscle fibres were larger in deep than in superficial samples. Bloomstrand and Ekblom (1982) have shown that there is only a very small variation in fibre size and distribution indices in normal subjects subjected to repeated biopsies of the quadriceps (vastus lateralis) muscle. Further, they noted that there was concordance between the two legs in individual subjects.

The standard deviation of the mean fibre diameter in normal muscle is usually less than 10 μm. Another quantitative method for expressing variability in fibre diameter, suggested by Brooke and Engel (1969), uses weighting factors to indicate the presence of fibres larger or smaller than those within the normal range; that is 40–80 μm in adult men and 30–70 μm

Table 3.1 Normal mean muscle fibre diameters in adult biceps brachii (μm) from Brooke and Engel, 1969)

	Type 1	Type 2
Men	64	73
Women	57	47

in adult women. This method gives increased numerical weight to very large or to very small fibres, the result being expressed as hypertrophy factors or atrophy factors. Thus, in men fibres of 30–40 μm diameter are given a weight of 1 and fibres of 10–20 μm diameter a weight of 3. These weights are divided by the total number of fibres measured. The resulting number is multiplied by 1000 to produce an atrophy factor. A similar method is used to calculate the hypertrophy factor in the same muscle fibres.

A simpler method of showing fibre atrophy or hypertrophy is to construct fibre size histograms, expressed as a percentage of the total number of fibres measured. This histogram can be compared visually, or by subtraction, with normal muscle biopsies from the same muscles.

All these methods are time consuming and rarely contribute to diagnosis, although they are useful in research, for example in studies of disuse atrophy or exercise-induced hypertrophy of muscle fibres. Computer-assisted methods of planimetry for measuring fibre area are also available; these usually involve the observer in tracing the outline of muscle fibres on to a graphics tablet linked to a microcomputer, using a drawing tube attached to the microscope. The value of these measurements in relation to fibre diameter measurements remains to be established (see Slavin et al., 1982).

3.2 Fibre-type distribution

Muscle fibres are distributed in a mosaic pattern of the different fibre types, the mosaic approximately conforming to a random distribution. The muscle fibres making up individual motor units are distributed over a wide cross-sectional area of any muscle, so that individual muscle fibres

---

Fig. 3.2 (a) Adult muscle × 140; ATPase, pH 4.6. There is a mosaic distribution of Type 1 (dark), Type 2A (pale) and Type 2B (intermediate) fibres, with approximately equal numbers of fibres of each type. This muscle is normal, apart from the presence of a few, isolated, small Type 1 fibres. The interfascicular planes can be clearly recognized. (b) Infant muscle (aged 2 years). × 237; ATPase, pH 4.6. The three fibre types are well developed, but the muscle fibres are very much smaller than in the adult. The fascicular pattern can be clearly seen.

in a motor unit are located in many different fascicles (see Fig. 1.1). It is unusual for more than two or three muscle fibres within a motor unit to be in contact with each other (Edstrom and Kugelberg, 1968); most such fibres are not situated in apposition with each other in normal muscle. The mosaic pattern of normal muscle thus consists of many different intermingled motor units each made up of fibres of one of the three major histochemical types. However, this relationship depends, to some extent, on the relative predominance of a particular fibre type within a muscle. For example, the soleus muscle contains predominantly Type 1 fibres and in this muscle the Type 1 fibres therefore often appear close to each other. This is particularly prominent when 70% or more fibre-type predominance is present. In most muscles Type 2 fibres predominate; in the most commonly biopsied muscles, the biceps brachii, deltoid and quadriceps, there are twice as many Type 2 as Type 1 fibres. However, in these muscles there are similar proportions of Type 2A, Type 2B and Type 1 muscle fibres.

The relative predominance of the different fibre types is, to some extent, an inherited characteristic. Some people tend to have more Type 1 fibres than others (Komi et al., 1977), a characteristic likely to lead to particular abilities in endurance athletic events. Training for endurance events may produce a relative increase in the proportion of Type 2B fibres (Jansson and Kaijser, 1977) and in weight-lifters trained for sudden maximal contraction of muscles these fibres may show selective hypertrophy (Saltin et al., 1976).

3.3   Fibre-type predominance

In normal muscle Type 1 muscle fibres constitute less than 55% of the fibres in a biopsy (Fig. 2.3), and Type 2 muscle fibres less than 80% (Dubowitz and Brooke, 1973). Predominance of Type 1 or Type 2 fibres is thus said to occur if these figures (Fig. 3.3) are exceeded (see Chapter 4).

3.4   Histological features

Several other features of normal muscle can be quantified and these are useful measures of normality.

3.4.1   Central nucleation

In transverse section each muscle fibre contains one or more subsarcolemmal nuclei. Normal muscle fibres contain less than 8 such nuclei (Greenfield et al., 1957). Centrally located nuclei are found in less than 3% of normal muscle fibres (Greenfield et al., 1957).

Fig. 3.3 × 380; ATPase pH 9.5. Fibre-type predominance. There is a relative excess of Type 1 fibres. Type 2 fibre atrophy is also a feature of this biopsy.

3.4.2   Fat and fibrous tissue

The interfascicular planes of normal muscle consist of connective and fibrous tissue, but in most biopsies this plane of tissue is thin. Most muscles also contain thick fibrous planes acting as internal tendons or sites of insertion of muscle fibres but these should not normally be included in a biopsy. The larger interfascicular boundaries may contain some fatty tissue but this is an uncommon feature of normal muscle, and fatty tissue does not infiltrate or replace muscle fibres themselves in normal biopsies.

The endomysium is thin and barely discernible in young people, but thickens slightly with increasing age (Rubinstein, 1960; Swash and Fox, 1972a). This endomysial tissue is not normally thick enough to cause more than very slight separation of muscle fibres from each other.

3.4.3   Fibre splitting

In normal muscle, fibre splitting is found only at the tendinous insertion of muscle fibres (Bell and Conen, 1968). This can be recognized by the proximity of these split fibres to bands of collagenous tissue. Fibre splitting may also occur in normal subjects following training, when it represents a response accompanying work-induced hypertrophy (Edgerton, 1970; Hall-Craggs, 1970). Regenerating and necrotic fibres are not found in normal muscle.

3.4.4   Muscle spindles

Muscle spindles occur in all human skeletal muscles except the facial muscles and the diaphragm (Fig. 3.4). The fibrous capsule of the spindle encloses 4–14 intrafusal muscle fibres in a mucopolysaccharide-filled periaxial space (Swash and Fox, 1972a). These intrafusal muscle fibres are smaller than adult extrafusal muscle fibres but larger than the extrafusal muscle fibres of infants. The intrafusal muscle fibres have complex enzyme histochemical reactions, which differ in the two main types of fibre, the larger nuclear bag and the smaller nuclear chain fibres (for review see Swash, 1982). Spindles are more frequently found in motor point biopsies than at other sites in individual muscles. Most spindles occur close to neurovasular bundles in the interfascicular plane.

Golgi tendon organs occur in tendinous septa; they are rarely found in muscle biopsies. Occasionally Pacinian corpuscles are seen in muscle, usually in close relation to muscle spindles.

Muscle spindles and Golgi tendon organs can be recognized in transverse or longitudinal sections of muscle, either at biopsy or at autopsy. At autopsy gold chloride or silver nitrate block impregnation techniques have been used to demonstrate the innervation of muscle spindles in whole mounts (Fig. 3.5), but this is a specialized technique requiring microdissection or teasing using a stereo microscope (Swash and Fox, 1972b)

3.4.5   Nerves

Small nerve bundles are almost always seen in open muscle biopsies, and frequently in needle biopsies. They are found in the perifascicular regions in association with blood vessels, forming the *neurovascular bundles*. Smaller branches can rarely be recognized without silver impregnations. The nerve bundles contain myelinated fibres of various diameters, including motor axons innervating extrafusal and intrafusal muscle fibres, the alpha and gamma motor fibres, respectively, and large sensory axons innervating sensory receptors in muscle spindles, Golgi tendon organs and Pacinian capsules. Small C fibres mediating pain are also present.

Fig. 3.4 Muscle spindle in transverse section. × 560. (a) The spindle capsule, periaxial space and intrafusal muscle fibres can be seen. These fibres are much smaller than the extrafusal skeletal muscle fibres themselves. (b) ATPase, pH 9.4. There are three histochemical types of intrafusal muscle fibre in this reaction; darkly, intermediate, and lightly reactive fibres. The capsule is virtually non-reactive. It is important to recognize that these isolated small muscle fibres are normal structures.

Fig. 3.5 (a) Muscle spindle × 350. Teased Barker and Ip silver impregnation to demonstrate the pattern of sensory innervation in a de-efferented baboon spindle. The primary sensory ending is to the right, and the secondary to the left of the illustration. (b) Muscle spindle × 140. Teased Barker and Ip silver impregnation. The motor and sensory nerve fibres in this human spindle form a

complex distribution of endings on the intrafusal muscle fibres. Note the capillaries running across the microscope field. The thicker sensory nerve fibres and the fine gamma efferent (motor) fibres can be recognized. (c) Pacinian corpuscle. × 550; HE TS. Biopsy of a floppy child. Pacinian corpuscles are only rarely seen in muscle biopsies. (d) Pacinian corpuscle. Silver impregnation; teased preparation × 140. The central part of the receptor contains the sensory nerve fibre, sensitive to pressure deformation.

Fig. 3.6 EM × 44 100. Human motor end-plate. The presynaptic, axonal part of the end-plate contains clear, small vesicles (containing acetyl choline). The synapse itself consists of primary and secondary synaptic clefts lined by basement membrane. M, muscle, A, axon.

3.4.6 Blood vessels

In the neurovascular bundles small arteries and veins may be found. Within individual fascicles smaller vessels, consisting of arterioles, venules and perimysial capillaries can be identified. Each muscle fibre is surrounded by 2 to 5 capillaries (Andersson and Henriksson, 1977).

3.4.7 Motor end-plates

Each muscle fibre is in contact with a single motor end-plate. The neuromuscular junction consists of a neural component and a muscular component, but this detail can only be clearly seen with the electron microscope (Fig. 3.6). With the light microscope the soleplate or muscular part of the end-plate consists of a slight elevation of the surface of the muscle fibre often associated with a few 'soleplate nuclei' to form the Doyère eminence. The neural part of the end-plate is separated from the muscle fibre by the synaptic cleft, and consists of short axonal expansions, covered by Schwann cell cytoplasm. This cleft consists of complex, closely apposed synaptic folds in which acetylcholinesterase can be demonstrated. The axonal expansions contain mitochondria and multiple clear synaptic vesicles. Differences between motor end-plates innervating Type 1 and Type 2 muscle fibres have been described (Duchen, 1971) but these cannot readily be recognized without quantitative ultrastructural studies.

Most muscle biopsies do not contain motor end-plates, since it is not common for muscle biopsies to be routinely taken from the region of the end-plate zone, i.e., at the motor point of the muscle. The supravital methylene blue method has been much used to demonstrate the terminal axonal pattern, and the structure of the neural part of the motor end-plates, the subneural apparatus, in research studies of neuro-muscular disorders, especially in myasthenia gravis (Coërs and Woolf, 1959).

References

Andersson, P. and Henriksson, J. (1977), Capillary supply of the quadriceps femoris muscle of man: Adaptive response to exercise. *J. Physiol. (Lond.)* **270**, 677–90.
Bell, C. D. and Conen, P. E. (1968), Histopathological changes in Duchenne muscular dystrophy. *J Neurol. Sci.*, **7**, 529–44.
Bloomstrand, E. and Ekblom, B. (1982), The needle biopsy technique for fibre type determination in human skeletal muscle – a methodological study. *Acta Physiol. Scand*; **116**, 437–42.

Brooke, M. H. and Engel, W. K (1969), The histographic analysis of human muscle biopsies with regard to fibre types. 1. Adult male and female. *Neurology (Minn.)* **19**, 221–33.

Coërs, C. and Woolf, A. L. (1959), *The Innervation of Muscle: a biopsy study*, Blackwell Scientific Publications, Oxford.

Dubowitz, V. and Brooke, M. H. (1973), *Muscle Biopsy – a modern approach*, W. B. Saunders London.

Duchen, L. W. (1971), An electron microscope comparison of motor end-plates of slow and fast skeletal muscle fibres of the mouse. *J. Neurol. Sci.*, **14**, 37–45.

Edgerton, V. R. (1970), Morphology and histochemistry of the soleus muscle from normal and exercised rats. *Am. J. Anat.*, **127**, 81–7.

Edstrom, L. and Kugelberg, E. (1968), Histochemical composition, distribution of fibres and fatiguability of single motor units. *J. Neurol. Neurosurg. Psychiatry*, **31**, 424–33.

Greenfield, J. G., Shy, G. M., Alvord, E. C. and Berg, L. (1957), *An Atlas of Muscle Pathology in Neuromuscular Diseases*, Churchill Livingstone, Edinburgh.

Hall-Craggs, E. C. B. (1970), The longitudinal division of fibres in overloaded rat skeletal muscle. *J. Anat.*, **107**, 459–70.

Jansson, E. and Kaijser, L. (1977), Muscle adaptation to extreme endurance training in man. *Acta Physiol. Scand.*, **100**, 315–24.

Komi P. V., Viitasalo, J. H. T., Havu, M. *et al.* (1977), Skeletal muscle fibres and muscle enzyme activities in monozygous and dizygous twins of both sexes. *Acta Physiol. Scand.*, **100**, 385–92.

Polgar, J., Johnson, M. A., Weightman, D. and Appleton, D. (1973), Data on fibre size in thirty-six human muscles: an autopsy study. *J. Neurol. Sci.*, **19**, 307–18.

Rubinstein, L. F. (1960), Ageing changes in muscle. In *Structure and Function of Muscle*, Vol. 3 (ed. G. H. Bourne), Academic Press, London, Ch. 7, pp. 209–26.

Saltin, B., Nazar, K., Costill, D. C. *et al.* (1976), The nature of the training response: peripheral and central adaptations to one-legged exercise. *Acta Physiol. Scand.*, **96**, 289–305.

Slavin, G., Sowter, C., Ward, P. and Paton, K. (1982), Measurement of striated muscle fibre diameters using interactive computer-aided microscopy. *J. Clin. Pathol.*, **35**, 1268–71.

Swash, M. (1982), Muscle spindle pathology. In *Skeletal Muscle Pathology* (Eds F. Mastaglia and J. N. Walton), Churchill Livingstone, Edinburgh.

Swash, M. and Fox, K. P., (1972a), The effect of age on human skeletal muscle: studies of the morphology and innervation of muscle spindles. *J. Neurol. Sci.*, **16**, 417–32.

Swash, M. and Fox, K. P. (1972b), Techniques for the demonstration of human muscle spindle innervation in neuromuscular disease. *J. Neurol. Sci.*, **15**, 291–302.

4 Histological features of myopathic and neurogenic disorders

It is usually not difficult to decide whether a muscle biopsy is normal or abnormal. Minor abnormalities such as slight changes in fibre size, or a slight increase in central nucleation, which may only be recognized by morphometric and statistical analysis, are not generally important in diagnosis, unless they are accompanied by other, more obvious changes. However, in some conditions, such as McArdle's disease, the routine histological and enzyme histochemical techniques may not reveal any striking abnormality, the diagnosis being recognized only when special techniques are applied. It is not appropriate, or economic, to try to investigate every biopsy with a complete range of histochemical techniques. A decision as to how far to pursue the investigation must be made on the basis of clinical information and the results of laboratory tests, in addition to the findings on the routine histological and enzyme histological methods. Histological abnormalities almost invariably accompany weakness.

The clinical findings and the results of laboratory and electrophysiological tests usually indicate whether the patient's muscular symptoms, especially weakness, are due to myopathic or neurogenic disease, but difficulties often arise in the investigation of patients with proximal muscular weakness. In these patients the distinction can only be made by muscle biopsy (Black *et al.*, 1974). The abnormalities found in myopathic and neurogenic disorders overlap to some extent, and this can lead to difficulties if enzyme histochemical techniques are not used. The recent recognition of the frequency of spinal muscular atrophy in patients presenting with proximal weakness stems from use of these newer methods. Formerly, most of these patients were considered to be suffering from limb–girdle muscular dystrophy. Despite these areas of overlap there are certain cardinal features of myopathic and neurogenic disorders and these are of great importance in diagnosis.

The first step in diagnosis, having recognized that a muscle biopsy is abnormal, is to decide whether the abnormality is *myopathic* or *neurogenic*;

47

this decision can only be made with certainty after study of the enzyme histochemical techniques, particularly the NADH and ATPase preparations.

4.1   Myopathic disorders

The main histological features of myopathic disorders are shown in Table 4.1. The general features shown in this table are abnormalities characteristic of myopathies, especially in inherited muscular dystrophies and inflammatory or toxic myopathies. In metabolic myopathies, on the other hand, fibre necrosis and regeneration are relatively uncommon, although other features, especially Type 2 fibre atrophy, central nucleation and increased variability in fibre size may be present. Many myopathies, especially the benign myopathies of childhood, are recognized by the occurrence of specific morphological changes within muscle fibres, and these may be virtually the only abnormality in the biopsy. These specific abnormalities will be discussed in later chapters.

Table 4.1 Histological features of myopathies

General features
   Single fibre necrosis, and regeneration
   Increased variability in fibre size, including hypertrophy and/or atrophy
   Increased central nucleation
   Selective Type 2 fibre atrophy
   Type 1 fibre predominance
   Fibre splitting
   Endomysial fibrosis and fat replacement of muscle fibres
   Changes in myofibrillar pattern e.g. whorled fibres and moth-eaten fibres
   Fibre-type grouping uncommon

Features specific to certain myopathies
   Perivascular and endomysial mononuclear cell infiltration
   Perifascicular atrophy
   Various specific morphological abnormalities in muscle fibres e.g. hyaline fibres, rod bodies, ragged-red fibres, central cores, tubular aggregates
   Abnormalities in blood vessels
   Muscle spindle abnormalities, e.g. myotonic dystrophy

4.1.1   Muscle fibre necrosis

Necrosis is a common and fundamental feature of many myopathies. It may result from a variety of factors, including trauma, heat, cold, vascular insufficiency, drugs and toxins, and all these factors have been used experimentally to study the initial histological features of necrosis and the sequence of regenerative changes that follow. The well-known descriptions of muscle fibre necrosis, consisting of vacuolation, hyaline changes, and Zenker's waxy degeneration (Zenker, 1864), are based on the appearances seen in paraffin-embedded material. In frozen sections the histological features differ somewhat from this pattern, largely because of the absence of fixation artefact.

A sequence of changes occurs in necrotic fibres (Figs 4.1 and 4.2). The earliest abnormality recognizable by light microscopy is a loss of granularity, producing an amorphous eosinophilic appearance in HE preparations (Fig. 4.1). At this stage the ATPase reactivity is unchanged, since myofibrils remain *in situ*, but with SDH or NADH the fibre appears either less reactive than normal, due to loss of mitochondrial enzymes, or appears floccular. Later, areas of patchy pallor can be seen in HE preparations. This is accompanied by pallor of nuclei and by the appearance of DNA in the sarcoplasm; acid phosphatase and RNA can usually also be demonstrated at this time. Infiltration by macrophages follows, usually leaving the basement membrane intact. Regeneration (see below) then begins.

Fig. 4.1 × 427; HE. Necrosis of this fibre has proceeded to macrophage infiltration of the abnormal part of the fibre. The ultrastructural counterpart of this phase of fibre necrosis is shown in Fig. 4.6.

Segmental necrosis is a term used to refer to necrosis of only part of a fibre. This can sometimes be recognized in single transverse sections, but is more usually seen in longitudinal sections. When necrosis results from vascular factors, or from 'toxic' effects, as in some drug-induced myopathies, e.g. that due to epsilon amino caproic acid (Swash and Schwartz, 1983) widespread simultaneous necrosis of many muscle fibres

Fig. 4.2 × 560; HE. (a) This fibre shows a floccular appearance with plump nuclei. This probably represents regeneration following necrosis. (b) In this longitudinal section the necrotic fibre also contains several early regenerating myoblasts. (c) × 6000; EM. Necrotic fibre adjacent to normal fibre. The disarrayed myofibrils and mitochondria may represent an early stage of regeneration.

may occur (Fig. 4.3). The basement membrane and endomysium is usually unaffected in this form of necrosis, so that empty, or macrophage-filled endomysial tubes remain (subendomysial necrosis).

In other myopathies, especially muscular dystrophies, and polymyositis, necrotic fibres are found scattered through the biopsy or in clusters in different parts of the biopsy. Infiltration of necrotic fibres by macrophages requires adequate capillary perfusion. In some cases of inflammatory myopathies this does not occur and in this situation necrotic muscle fibres may remain more or less intact, but show marked loss of enzyme activity. These are sometimes called *ghost fibres* (Fig. 4.4).

Hyaline fibres have been considered as a special type of muscle fibre type necrosis but it has also been suggested that this abnormality, which is a particularly prominent feature of Duchenne muscular dystrophy (Fig. 4.5), is due to localized hypercontraction.

Fig. 4.5 × 405; HE. Duchenne muscular dystrophy. The large, rounded intensely eosinophilic fibres in this paraffin-embedded section have undergone hyaline change.

Ultrastructural studies of muscle fibre necrosis have revealed that mitochondrial changes are marked in the early stages. The myofilaments degenerate later, forming amorphous masses of electron-dense material, and the sarcolemmal tubular system becomes disorganized. During macrophage ingestion the myofilaments tend to become broken into small pieces, consisting of A band material; Z and I band material cannot be identified (Fig. 4.6). This is a feature of necrosis following damage to the fibre's plasma membrane (Cullen and Fulthorpe, 1982). Initially myofilamentous breakdown and loss may be focal within a fibre.

Fig. 4.3 Acute myopathy due to epsilon amino caproic acid. × 380; HE. Widespread floccular necrosis of muscle fibres, with continuous regeneration occurring from subendomysial crescents, probably representing a satellite cell origin for the regeneration (see Kennard *et al.* (1980)).
Fig. 4.4 × 350; HE. Chronic polymyositis. The 'ghost' fibre (arrow) is pale and amorphous, and contains pale nuclei, probably those of macrophages; these are features of necrosis.

Fig. 4.6   EM × 8750. Polymyositis. The necrotic fibre contains a macrophage (M) within its sarcoplasm. This cell contains electron dense lysosomal inclusions, and it lacks a basement membrane. The myofilaments are broken up into A band segments (A), and Z and I band material is absent. Outside the fibre, fibroblast cell processes (F) and capillaries (C) are seen.

4.1.2   Muscle fibre regeneration

Regeneration occurs after necrosis or injury in most tissues of the body and muscle fibres, which are particularly susceptible to injury in everyday life, have considerable regenerative potential. In muscle biopsies it is common to find both necrotic and regenerating fibres in close proximity, indicating that degeneration and repair are occurring concurrently.

Regenerative changes. After fibre necrosis, regeneration can occur either in continuity with the undamaged portions of the fibre ('continuous' repair) or from myoblast formation in the necrotic segment itself ('discontinuous' repair). Regeneration begins at a stage when phagocytosis of necrotic material is still incomplete. At this time mononucleated cells are still abundant in the interstitium around the necrotic fibre.

In 'continuous' regeneration, surviving muscle nuclei become enlarged and vesicular about 4 days after injury, and migrate to the centre of the fibre. The surrounding cytoplasm becomes basophilic, losing its striations and by the 5th–10th day after injury ribbons of basophilic, foamy non-striated sarcoplasm can be seen in the necrotic segment. In 'discontinuous' regeneration, regeneration proceeds from mononucleated myoblasts. These form a component of the basophilic fusiform cells found along the inner surface of the basement membrane of necrotic muscle fibres. Several days after injury these cells form long basophilic multinucleated ribbons which later fuse, forming a new fibre. These ribbons of differentiating sarcoplasm are similar to the myotubes formed during embryonic myogenesis.

The origin of myoblasts during regeneration is controversial (Fig. 4.7). They could arise by segregation from the damaged myofibre itself, by activation of satellite cells pre-existing in the sarcolemmal sheath, or by metaplasia from circulating mesenchymal cells. The weight of evidence (Resnik, 1973) favours the first and second of these suggestions. In particular, the role of satellite cells in regeneration after injury has received support from the observation of activation of these cells after a variety of experimental and naturally occurring modes of fibre injury. Satellite cells are found in normal muscle fibres as a nucleus, surrounded by sparse granular sarcoplasm containing abundant free ribosomes, Golgi apparatus, endoplasmic reticulum and mitochondria, but devoid of any myofilaments. The satellite cell is limited by plasma membrane, and is situated beneath the basement membrane of the muscle fibre. The numbers of such cells in muscle are increased after injury (Resnik, 1973) and after denervation (Ontell, 1974). Resnik (1973) has reviewed the ultrastructural sequence of changes giving rise to myoblast formation in these cells during regeneration after cold-induced injury.

Webb (1977) has drawn attention to the importance of programmed cell death of myotubes during embryonic myogenesis. The stimulus for cell death is unknown, but a similar phenomenon probably occurs during differentiation of myoblasts in regenerative repair, since large numbers of developing myotubes are found in the early stages of repair, before fusion occurs and the single myofibre is reconstituted. It is possible that the

Fig. 4.7 EM regeneration. Acute dermatomyositis of adult onset. (a) × 7200. Regeneration from satellite cells results in myoblast formations so that several maturing muscle fibres appear enclosed by a single sarcolemmal tube (basal lamina) although each has its own plasma membrane tube. The nuclei show a

dispersed chromatin pattern and the myofibrils are contained in a granular sarcoplasm. Variations in maturity of myofibrillar development are apparent. (b) × 8400. Regenerating myofilamentous material is not yet orientated in the long axis of this fibre.

achievement of functional reinnervation, which can only occur when the fibre is reconstituted across the necrotic segment, is important in this process (Fig. 4.8).

In muscle biopsies regenerating fibres have a characteristic appearance (Fig. 4.8). The sarcoplasm appears basophilic and granular, and it often contains copious small lipid droplets. The sarcoplasmic nuclei are usually large and vesicular with prominent nucleoli and a dispersed chromatin pattern. The myofibrillar density is low so that myofibrillar enzymes, such as the myofibrillar ATPase may be poorly reactive, and fibre typing may be difficult since these fibres often show intermediate properties in the ATPase reactions. The basophilic sarcoplasm of regenerating fibres shows increased RNA content, and increased acid phosphatase activity (Neerunjun and Dubowitz, 1977). Sometimes these changes are seen in only part of the transverse diameter of a fibre. Regenerating fibres often occur in small groups and, even if single, they are usually smaller than normal fibres.

4.1.3   Increased variability in fibre size

In normal muscle most muscle fibres are 40–80 μm in diameter in men, and 30–70 μm in diameter in women (see Chapter 3). It is characteristic of myopathic disorders that many fibres, larger or smaller than the normal range, occur in the biopsy and in some disorders, for example in limb-girdle muscular dystrophy, very large (>120 μm) and very small (<20 μm) fibres may occur. Histograms of fibre diameter in such biopsies demonstrate the wide range of diameters. This increased variability in fibre size is due to hypertrophy, probably occurring as a compensatory response to the increased load imposed on surviving healthy muscle fibres in muscles in which loss of functioning muscle fibres has occurred (Swash and Schwartz, 1977), and to atrophy. Atrophy results from incomplete regeneration, from necrosis, or from fibre splitting. Increased variability in fibre size may be the most striking abnormality in relatively mild non-progressive myopathies; this often reflects selective atrophy of a fibre type, usually of Type 2 fibres as in many metabolic myopathies.

Fig. 4.8   Regeneration (a) × 380; HE. Regenerating subendomysial myoblasts have differentiated but have not yet fused to form single new fibres. The perimysium separates a regenerating fascicle from an adjacent nearly normal fascicle in this patient with acute polymyositis (see also Fig. 5.1b). (b) × 380; ATPase, pH 4.3. Serial section to (a). The regenerating subendomysial fibre clusters are clearly seen. Some fibres are of intermediate type (Type 2C).

Fig. 4.9 × 350; PAS. The fibre in the middle of the field contains two centrally-placed nuclei, and another fibre contains a single centrally-placed nucleus.

Fig. 4.10 × 350; HE. Polymyositis. These hypertrophied fibres, greater than 100 μm diameter, contain multiple central nuclei. There is a moderate increase in the amount of endomysial fibrous tissue.

4.1.4   Increased central nucleation

Central nucleation is common in myopathies (Fig. 4.9). It usually occurs in hypertrophied fibres but it is also found in small basophilic regenerating fibres (Fig. 4.10). In hypertrophied fibres multiple central nuclei are often seen, and these are sometimes associated with clefts or splits in the sarcoplasm of the fibre. Multiple central nucleation in fibres of normal size is a feature of myotonic dystrophy. In normal muscle up to 3% of the fibres may contain central nuclei.

4.1.5   Selective Type 2 fibre atrophy

In myopathies selective atrophy of Type 2 fibres is a common finding (Fig. 4.11). However, this is not a specific feature of myopathies since it is found also in disuse atrophy, in patients with stroke and in Parkinson's disease. Occasionally, especially in steroid myopathy, Type 2 atrophy may be so marked that the atrophic fibres appear thin and pointed, resembling acute denervation. Unless ATPase preparations are made this selective involvement cannot be recognized. In most myopathies the Type 2B fibres are more atrophic than the Type 2A fibres.

4.1.6   Type 1 fibre predominance

Fibre-type predominance is not in itself a specific abnormality, and the selection implied in small needle biopsies may make it difficult to assess.

Fig. 4.11   × 140; ATPase. Steroid myopathy. The dark Type 2 fibres are atrophic; and the pale Type 1 fibres are of normal size.

However, Type 1 fibre predominance (>55% Type 1 fibres) is, in general, associated with myopathies, particularly Duchenne dystrophy and childhood myopathies. It is also found in about a third of biopsies from patients with limb–girdle muscular dystrophy.

When a biopsy contains a large proportion of fibres of one histochemical type caution must be exercised in assessing whether or not there is fibre-type grouping, since fibres of a single type will inevitably be found in proximity to each other (Johnson *et al.*, 1973). Fibre-type grouping can only be recognized with certainty when groups of both Type 1 and Type 2 fibres occur.

Fig. 4.12 Fibre splitting. (a) × 560; NADH. A cleft of splitting invaginates the large fibre and almost bisects it. This process is often associated with a centrally-located nucleus. (b) × 120; HE. Serial sections 80 μm apart to show the relation of fibre splitting to central nuclei. (c) EM × 14 250. Longitudinal section. A cleft lined by plasma membrane and basement membrane invaginates the fibre, directed downward toward the nucleus.

(c)

4.1.7   Fibre splitting

Hypertrophied fibres are particularly likely to show fibre splitting (Fig. 4.12). The split usually begins at the periphery of the fibre and is directed toward a centrally located nucleus, but in some instances the split may consist solely of a central cleft associated with nearby nuclei. The cleft at the edges of the frank zone of splitting is usually basophilic and the nuclei associated with this cleft appear vesicular. Sometimes a fibre may be split into multiple fragments. Fibre splitting is a normal phenomenon near musculo-tendinous insertions and it must not be confused with subendomysial regeneration which occurs in association with fibre necrosis. Muscle fibre splitting is a common feature of muscular dystrophies and it is also found in chronic polymyositis. It may also be a feature of long-standing neurogenic disorders in which secondary myopathic changes have developed (Schwartz *et al.*, 1976). *Ring fibres* can be interpreted as a special example of splitting in which one or more myofibrils become displaced from their normal longitudinal orientation to take up a spirally arranged location around the main group of myofibrils (Fig. 4.13).

4.1.8   Endomysial fibrosis and fatty replacement

These features represent a feature of the advanced stages of myopathic disease. Marked fibrosis is especially prominent in Duchenne muscular dystrophy, and fatty replacement of muscular tissue represents the late stages of disease, when compensatory processes have failed and regenerative repair no longer occurs.

4.1.9   Features specific to certain myopathies

These are described in relation to the disorder in which they are the predominant feature.

4.2   Neurogenic disorders

The main histological features of neurogenic disorders are shown in Table 4.2. In neurogenic disorders the histological features are not specific for particular disorders, since the changes in the muscle are themselves due to loss of innervation (*denervation*) or to *reinnervation* after denervation.

Fig. 4.13 Ring fibres (a) × 560; NADH. Two small fibres show displaced, peripherally-located myofibrils. This is a non-specific abnormality. (b) EM × 15000. Myotonic dystrophy. A ring-like displaced myofibril encircles the fibre.

Table 4.2 Histological features of neurogenic disorders

Denervation
  Disseminated neurogenic atrophy
  Target fibres
  Grouped neurogenic atrophy
  Changes in intramuscular nerve bundles

Reinnervation
  Fibre-type grouping
  Fibre-type predominance

Neurogenic disorders may be acute or chronic and many of the latter may continue for many years; for example the familial neuropathies and spinal muscular atrophies. In these long-standing neurogenic disorders secondary myopathic changes may develop in affected muscles, in addition to neurogenic changes.

4.2.1   Histological features of denervation

After denervation muscle fibres undergo atrophy. This atrophy is a slow process reaching its peak in about 4 months after interruption to the nerve supply. In most neurogenic disorders, however, denervation is neither total nor of abrupt onset. Rather, the disease is progressive and of gradual onset, so that muscle fibres belonging to one motor unit in a muscle may be denervated while muscle fibres forming part of an adjacent motor unit may still have a normal innervation. There is thus a wide variation in the state of innervation, and in the stage of the neurogenic process in individual muscles. The histological appearances in neurogenic disorders reflect these processes.

After nerve section the first change in a muscle is increased roundness of the sarcolemmal nuclei, which develop prominent nucleoli. After about 2 weeks an increase in central nucleation is evident. Reduction in muscle fibre diameter becomes detectable after about 4 weeks and after 2 months the muscle fibre diameter is reduced to about half normal. The striations, however, are still present. Atrophy reaches its peak between the third and fourth months after denervation, and these muscle fibres tend to assume a polygonal or pointed shape at about this stage, or later. At this late stage, i.e. more than 6 months after denervation, the muscle fibres are small (<20 µm diameter) and the sarcolemmal nuclei are small, dark and pyknotic (Adams *et al.*, 1953). Even after nerve section, however, some muscle fibres are relatively more resistant to denervation atrophy than others. Target fibres are a special feature of acute denervation (see below).

(a) *Disseminated neurogenic atrophy*. The minimal detectable abnormality in a neurogenic disorder, using histological techniques, consists of single atrophic muscle fibres, or small clusters of atrophic fibres, found scattered through the biopsy (Fig. 4.14). These atrophic fibres appear thin and pointed, and react strongly in NADH preparations so that they appear abnormally dark with this technique (Fig. 4.15). They also react positively in non-specific esterase preparations. With myofibrillar ATPase they may be of either major histochemical type. They usually contain dark, pyknotic nuclei and these may be multiple in a single cross-section. They do not show marked acid phosphatase activity and they are not basophilic.

These atrophic fibres represent muscle fibres denervated by damage to a single motor axon or to its terminal twigs. They are therefore found in muscle biopsies both in anterior horn cell diseases, and in motor neuropathies.

(b) *Grouped neurogenic atrophy*. This consists of groups of small atrophic fibres, of the same histochemical type in myofibrillar ATPase preparations (Fig. 4.16). The fibres in each group are generally of similar size and may represent part or the whole of a fascicle. The individual atrophic fibres in grouped neurogenic atrophy (Fig. 4.16b) show the same histological and histochemical features, particularly the prominent reactivity in SDH and NADH preparations, as do the atrophic fibres in disseminated neurogenic atrophy; they thus show the histological

Fig. 4.14 × 560; ATPase, pH 9.4. Two thin, pointed atrophic Type 2 fibres are surrounded by normal Type 1 and Type 2 fibres; *disseminated neurogenic atrophy*.

features of denervation. The significance of grouped denervation atrophy is that it implies that denervation has occurred after reinnervation (*see fibre-type grouping* below) and it is therefore a phenomenon representing a relatively decompensated, and later stage, of a progressive neurogenic disorder.

Fig. 4.15   × 560; NADH. The central narrow, darkly-reactive fibre contains a target zone consisting of a pale central area rimmed with positively reacting material; *target fibre abnormality*.

Fig. 4.16 (a) × 350; ATPase pH 9.4. In the centre of the field is a group of narrow atrophic fibres; *small grouped atrophy*. (b) EM × 4200. Two denervated fibres. Note the prominent nuclei and the sparse degenerate myofilamentous material. There is a capillary nearby.

(c) *Target fibres*. These consist of fibres containing abnormalities in their centres best seen in myofibrillar ATPase and NADH preparations (Fig. 4.17). The abnormality consists of a central, unstained zone surrounded by a densely stained intermediate zone and a third relatively normal outer zone extending to the edge of the fibre. Type 1 fibres are preferentially affected. Target fibres are found in acutely denervated muscle, especially in peripheral nerve lesions, such as nerve transections and acute neuropathies, but they may sometimes be found in rapidly progressive anterior horn cell disease, e.g. motor neuron disease. Although a characteristic feature of denervation they can be produced experimentally by tenotomy (Engel *et al.*, 1966).

Fig. 4.17 × 350; NADH. A group of atrophic, darkly-reactive fibres (*grouped denervation atrophy*) show target formations.

(d) *Changes in intramuscular nerve bundles*. Biopsies often contain intramuscular nerve bundles and, in the presence of marked neurogenic change, these nerve fascicles may themselves show abnormalities of diagnostic value. For example, Wallerian degeneration and Schwann cell hyperplasia can easily be recognized in axonal neuropathies and certain demyelinating neuropathies, respectively.

4.2.2 *Histological features of reinnervation*

Reinnervation after denervation may occur, in favourable circumstances, e.g. in acute neuropathies, by regeneration of axons to reinnervate the motor end-plates of the denervated fibres before severe and irreversible muscle fibre atrophy has occurred.

In most progressive neurogenic disorders, however, muscle fibre reinnervation occurs by collateral axonal sprouting from nearby axons representing the terminal neuronal tree of a different anterior horn cell from that originally innervating these muscle fibres (Wohlfart, 1957; 1958). Because of the intermingling of muscle fibres belonging to different motor units in the muscle, such collateral sprouts may be only a few hundred micrometers long. Further, collateral reinnervation may result in a muscle fibre receiving new innervation from a motor unit of different histochemical type, thus inducing this muscle fibre to change its histochemical type and resulting in enlargement of the residual motor units. As more fibres become reinnervated by this process, small groups of reinnervated fibres of the same histological type can be identified in the biopsy. Each reinnervated fibre receives innervation from a single axon, as in normal muscle.

Several factors prejudice the development of effective reinnervation. These include prominent muscle fibre atrophy prior to the arrival of collateral sprouts in the vicinity of the denervated fibres and failure of denervated fibres to receive collateral axonal sprouts either because of deficient capacity to sprout, due to metabolic abnormalities in neuronal or axonal cytoplasm, or because of physical factors in the muscle itself such as fibrous tissue barriers. Wohlfart (1957) estimated that collateral axonal sprouting is so effective that as many as 30% of anterior horn cells can be lost in motor neuron disease before weakness becomes clinically apparent. In such a muscle there would be marked histological evidence of reinnervation.

(a) *Fibre-type grouping*. In normal muscle the muscle fibres belonging to individual motor units are widely distributed within a limited area, up to 20%, of the cross-sectional area of a muscle, so that the fibres of individual motor units intermingle and their territories overlap (Edstrom and Kugelberg, 1968). Fibres belonging to a single motor unit are thus usually isolated but sometimes two or four such fibres are adjacent to each other, and occasionally up to six fibres occur together in a straight or curved row (Edstrom and Kugelberg, 1968). When reinnervation occurs by collateral axonal sprouting small or large groups of fibres of the same histochemical type are formed; *fibre-type grouping*. In experimental studies fibre-type grouping does not occur earlier than 6 weeks after peripheral nerve injury (Warszanski *et al.*, 1975).

The recognition of fibre-type grouping depends on somewhat arbitrary criteria. Fibre-type grouping is generally defined as the presence of two or more fibres of identical fibre type completely enclosed, at all points on their circumference, by other fibres of the same histochemical type

(Fig. 4.18). Since normal muscle fibres tend to be of approximately equal size, and to assume a six-sided configuration (see Willison, 1980) this definition implies that a group of fibres will contain not less than 10 fibres of the same histochemical type. However, the number of fibres required to produce fibre-type grouping will depend, to some extent, on the size of the fibres, particularly the size of the enclosed fibres themselves. If the latter are small, fewer surrounding fibres may be required to enclose them. It is thus an empirical criterion that a group should consist of at least 12 fibres before it can be regarded as significant. Furthermore, the presence of fibre-type grouping of both histochemical fibre types in the biopsy lends weight to the observation, and multiple areas of fibre-type grouping usually occur in well-established neurogenic disorders. A single zone of fibre-type grouping should be interpreted with caution since this may represent a nearby fascicle with a different proportion of one or other fibre type, and not fibre-type grouping.

Fig. 4.18 × 140; ATPase, pH 4.3. *Fibre-type grouping*. The central group consists of >12 fibres of the same histochemical type, and three of these fibres are entirely enclosed by fibres of the same type.

In muscles in which fibre-type predominance is marked it is difficult to recognize fibre-type grouping, unless the group consists of fibres of the less predominant type. Johnson *et al.* (1973) pointed out that two or more enclosed fibres will commonly occur when a fibre type is predominant by 70% or more.

In fibre-type grouping the fibres within the group usually vary in size, whereas in fibre-type predominance, they tend to be of more nearly uniform size.

(b) *Fibre-type predominance*. Fibre-type predominance may be a feature of neurogenic or myopathic conditions. Type 2 fibre predominance is often found in neurogenic disorders, whereas Type 1 fibre predominance is more frequently found in myopathies (Fig. 4.19). In a small biopsy fibre-type predominance may represent a sample of a large group of reinnervated fibres. This is a particular hazard of needle biopsies in which only a small sample of the muscle is available. When fibre-type predominance is found in a muscle such as vastus lateralis or biceps brachii, which normally contain approximately equal numbers of Type 1, Type 2A and Type 2B fibres, it assumes particular significance, and a neurogenic disorder should be suspected.

Fig. 4.19 × 140; ATPase, pH 4.3. *Fibre-type predominance*. The majority of the fibres in the field are of the same histochemical type. This appearance may, as in this example, resemble fibre-type grouping. One fibre, undergoing regeneration, appears fragmented.

4.2.3 *Secondary myopathic change in chronic neurogenic disorders*

In long-standing neurogenic disorders such as poliomyelitis, spinal muscular atrophy and hereditary motor neuropathies, histological changes resembling those of myopathies may be found. These myopathic changes pose a difficult problem in diagnosis since they may obscure the

Table 4.3 'Secondary myopathic' changes in chronic neurogenic disorders (see Cazzato, 1970; Drachman *et al.*, 1967; Haase and Shy, 1960; Schwartz *et al.*, 1976)

Histological evidence of denervation and reinnervation (see Table 4.2) plus:
Increased central nucleation
Longitudinal splitting of muscle fibres
Muscle fibre hypertrophy (mainly Type 1 fibres)
Degenerative changes
Isolated regenerating fibre clusters
Increased variation in fibre size
Interstitial fibrosis

---

underlying neurogenic lesion unless enzyme histochemical techniques are used to demonstrate the presence of denervated fibres, and fibre-type grouping. The most common myopathic features seen in these chronic neurogenic disorders are shown in Table 4.3. These changes occur as part of a sequence of compensatory phenomena in weakened muscles, particularly in relation to fibre hypertrophy and fibre splitting (Schwartz *et al.*, 1976; Swash and Schwartz, 1981).

References

Adams, R. D., Denny-Brown, D. and Pearson, C. M. (1953), *Diseases of Muscle*, Cassell, London.

Black, J. T., Bhatt, G. P., DeJesus, P. V. *et al.* (1974), Diagnostic accuracy of clinical data, quantitative electromyography and histochemistry in neuromuscular disease: a study of 105 cases. *J. Neurol. Sci.*, **21**, 59–70.

Cazzato, G. (1970), Myopathic changes in denervated muscle: a study of biopsy material in various neuromuscular diseases. In *Muscle Diseases* (eds J. N. Walton, N. Canal and G. Scarlato), Exerpta Medica, Amsterdam, pp. 392–401.

Cullen, M. J. and Fulthorpe, J. J. (1982), Phagocytosis of the A band following Z line and I band loss: Its significance in skeletal muscle breakdown. *J. Pathol.*, **138**, 129–43.

Drachman, D. B., Murphy, J. R. N., Nigam, M. P. and Hills, J. R. (1967), 'Myopathic' changes in chronically denervated muscle. *Arch. Neurol.*, **16**, 14–24.

Edstrom, L. and Kugelberg, E. (1968), Histochemical composition, distribution of fibres and fatiguability of single motor units. *J. Neurol. Neurosurg. Psychiatry*, **31** 424–33.

Engel, W. K., Brooke, M. H. and Nelson, P. G. (1966), Histochemical studies of denervated or tenotomised cat muscle. *Ann. NY Acad. Sci.*, **138**, 160–85.

Haase, G. R. and Shy, G. M. (1960), Pathological changes in muscle biopsies from patients with peroneal muscle atrophy. *Brain*, **83**, 631–7.

Johnson, M. A., Polgar, J., Weightman, D. and Appleton, D. (1973), Data on the distribution of fibre types in thirty six human muscles: an autopsy study. *J. Neurol. Sci.*, **18**, 111–29.

Neerunjun, S. J. S. and Dubowitz, V. (1977), Concomitance of basophilia, ribonucleic acid and acid phosphatase activity in regenerating muscle fibres. *J. Neurol. Sci.*, **33**, 95–109.

Ontell, M. (1974), Muscle satellite cells. *Anat. Rec.*, **178**, 211–28.
Resnik, M. (1973), Current concepts of skeletal muscle regeneration. In *The Striated Muscle* (ed. C. M. Pearson), Williams and Wilkins, Baltimore, pp. 185–225.
Schwartz, M. S., Sargeant, M. K. and Swash, M. (1976), Longitudinal fibre splitting in neurogenic muscular disorders – its relation to the pathogenesis of myopathic change. *Brain*, **99**, 617–36.
Swash, M. and Schwartz, M. S. (1977), Implications of longitudinal muscle fibre splitting in neurogenic and myopathic disorders. *J. Neurol. Neurosurg. Psychiatry*, **40**, 1152–9.
Swash, M. and Schwartz, M. S. (1981), *Neuromuscular Diseases: A Practical Approach to Diagnosis and Management*, Springer-Verlag, Berlin, Heidelberg, New York.
Swash, M. and Schwartz, M. S. (1983), Iatrogenic neuromuscular disorders: a review. *R. Soc. Med.*, **76**, 1414–51.
Warszanski, M., Telerman-Toppet, N., Durdu, J. *et al.* (1975), The early stages of neuromuscular regeneration after crushing the sciatic nerve in the rat. *J. Neurol. Sci.*, **24**, 21–32.
Webb, J. N. (1977), Cell death in developing skeletal muscle: histochemistry and ultrastructure. *J. Pathol.*, **123**, 175–80.
Willison, R. G. (1980), Arrangement of muscle fibres of a single motor unit in mammalian muscle. *Muscle Nerve*, **3**, 360–61.
Wohlfart, G. (1957), Collateral regeneration from residual motor nerve fibres in amyotrophic lateral sclerosis. *Neurology (Minneap.)* 7, 124–34.
Wohlfart, G. (1958), Collateral regeneration in partially denervated muscle. *Neurology (Minneap.)*, **8**, 175–80.
Zenker, F. A. (1864), Ueber die Veränderungen der Willkurlichen Muskeln im Typhus abdominalis. Vogel, Leipzig.

5   Inflammatory myopathies

Inflammatory myopathy is a common and complex problem. In our experience this is the presumptive diagnosis in nearly half the muscle biopsies sent to the laboratory. Accurate diagnosis of inflammatory myopathies is particularly important not only because treatment is possible, but because the unwanted effects of this treatment cannot lightly be disregarded.

There are a number of different varieties of inflammatory myopathy (Table 5.1). This classification is based on clinical associations (see Whitaker, 1982). However, in all these disorders the pathological features of inflammatory myopathy are found in the muscle biopsy. In some, for example sarcoid myopathy, or in infestations of muscle, e.g. trichinosis, certain additional specific features may be recognized, but the underlying inflammatory myopathy is the cornerstone of the diagnosis.

Table 5.1 Classification of inflammatory myopathies

Idiopathic polymyositis
Idiopathic dermatomyositis
Childhood-type dermatomyositis
Dermatomyositis or polymyositis associated with autoimmune disorders
    (a) Polyarteritis nodosa
    (b) Rheumatoid arthritis
    (c) Systemic lupus erythematosus
    (d) Scleroderma
    (e) Mixed connective tissue disease
    (f) Polymyalgia rheumatica and giant cell arteritis
    (g) Eosinophilic fasciitis with polymyositis
    (h) Polymyositis associated with myasthenia gravis
Dermatomyositis or polymyositis associated with malignancy
Sarcoid myopathy
Inclusion body polymyositis
Polymyositis due to infections
    (a) Viral and postinfection myositis
    (b) Bacterial myositis
    (c) Infestations of muscle

5.1 Clinical features of inflammatory myopathies

The disorder may present acutely or subacutely with painful and weak muscles, usually affecting proximal muscles more than distal but not necessarily symmetrically. Arthralgia, Raynaud's phenomenon, dysphagia, fever, lethargy, anorexia and weight loss are common features. In patients with cutaneous involvement a characteristic, violaceous, photosensitive skin rash affects the upper eyelids, cheeks, nose, knuckles, elbows and knees. The rash may precede or accompany muscular symptoms. The skin later becomes shiny and atrophic and the nail beds reddened. In some patients telangiectasia and nail bed infarcts, a feature of vasculitis, develop. In autoimmune disorders, polymyositis may be a presenting feature or, more commonly, a later development in the natural history of the disease. As a rule polymyositis in patients with rheumatoid arthritis, scleroderma, and systemic lupus erythematosus is relatively mild, but it may be more severe in polyarteritis nodosa. Symptoms usually outweigh pathological changes in muscle biopsies in polymyalgia rheumatica and giant cell arteritis. Sarcoid myopathy is an uncommon disorder usually more marked by pathological change than by symptoms.

5.2 Laboratory investigations

The creatine kinase (CK) is raised in most cases at diagnosis, and the ESR is increased in about half the cases. Other muscle enzymes can be detected in the blood, e.g. aldolase and pyruvate kinase. In severe, active cases myoglobinuria can be demonstrated. Tests for the detection of autoimmune disorders such as autoantibody titres, ESR, antinuclear factor and latex fixation tests, and plasma protein electrophoresis are most helpful in patients with recognized autoimmune syndromes, such as rheumatoid arthritis or systemic lupus erythematosus, but they may also show abnormalities in patients with polymyositis, particularly if there are features of mixed connective tissue disease. The ECG is abnormal in some patients with polymyositis but symptomatic cardiomyopathy is unusual. Investigations for occult neoplasms are generally unrewarding in patients under the age of 40 years without skin involvement.

5.3 Pathology

The changes found in muscle biopsies vary according to the severity and duration of the disease, and the effect of treatment, if any. Particularly characteristic abnormalities occur in the early stages of the illness (Table 5.2).

Table 5.2 Histological features of acute idiopathic polymyositis

---

Increased variability in fibre size
Atrophy of both fibre types
Increased central nucleation
'Moth-eaten' fibres
Angular atrophic fibres
Single fibre necrosis with phagocytosis
Regenerating basophilic fibres
Inflammatory cell infiltration
Perifascicular atrophy
Abnormalities usually locally distributed in the biopsy

5.3.1   Acute idiopathic polymyositis

In the early stages of the disease the muscle fibres tend to retain their polygonal shape, except in the peripheral zones of fibre atrophy, sometimes particularly prominent around the edges of fascicles; *perifascicular atrophy*. The latter is believed to result from ischaemia of fibres at the periphery of the fascicles. In some cases there are zones of muscle fibre necrosis within individual fascicles (Fig. 5.1) an appearance suggesting a vascular basis (Banker and Victor, 1966; Swash *et al.*, 1978). Fibre necrosis, with 'moth-eaten' architectural changes and endomysial oedema may be the most prominent abnormality at this stage of the disorder. Small denervated fibres, occurring in isolation or in small clusters may be a feature.

Inflammatory cell infiltrates are a major feature of most cases and are an important clue to diagnosis. They consist of aggregates of small lymphocytes together with macrophages, plasma cells and, occasionally, eosinophils. These cellular infiltrates may occur in relation to necrotic fibres or to small intra- or interfascicular blood vessels (Figs 5.1 and 5.2). In some biopsies focal cellular infiltrates are not found but in these cases there may be a diffuse increase in cellularity in the endomysium (Fig. 5.3). A diffuse increase in cellularity is also a feature of acute toxic myopathies in which muscle fibre necrosis has occurred, and focal inflammatory cell exudates may be a feature of some cases of facio-scapulo-humeral muscular dystrophy. They are therefore not absolutely diagnostic of

---

Fig. 5.1 (a) Acute childhood polymyositis, × 350; HE. A prominent focal lymphocytic infiltrate is situated in a muscle fascicle in relation to a thickened blood vessel (at the left edge of the illustration). Perifascicular atrophy is prominent but an adjoining fascicle (right) contains fibres of normal size. (b) × 60; ATPase, pH 4.3. Acute dermatomyositis. A zone of regenerating small fibres (to the left of the illustration) occupies several fascicles suggesting a vascular basis for fibre necrosis.

Fig. 5.2 × 350; HE. Acute polymyositis in an adult. The blood vessel is surrounded by lymphocytes and by a few plasma cells. The necrotic fibre is pale and contains macrophages. Several neighbouring fibres are smaller than normal and show enlarged, centrally-placed nuclei. These fibres are faintly basophilic, suggesting active regeneration.

Fig. 5.3 × 350; HE. Acute polymyositis. There is a sparse endomysial lymphocytic infiltrate varying in intensity in different parts of the biopsy. One fibre shows a necrotic segment.

inflammatory autoimmune polymyositis. Thrombosis and vasculitis are not commonly seen but, when present, are often focal. Fibrinoid necrosis of small vessels is very uncommon. Sometimes perivascular inflammatory cell infiltrates seem to be located near small veins rather than arterioles, a feature particularly found in the rare form of vasculitis described by Churg and Strauss (1951). Endomysial and interfascicular fibrosis, and areas of fat replacement are features only of chronic polymyositis.

In up to a quarter of muscle biopsies from patients with the clinical syndrome of acute idiopathic polymyositis, inflammatory cell infiltrates are absent. In these cases the diagnosis should be considered on the basis of the other histological features, especially the occurrence of active degeneration and regeneration, together with moth-eaten fibres (Fig. 5.4), perifascicular atrophy, and the focal distribution of the abnormality.

Fig. 5.4 × 350; NADH. Chronic polymyositis. Several fibres show a 'moth-eaten' appearance consisting of patchy areas of absent or normal enzyme activity. Note the variability in fibre size and the separation of the fibres, caused by thickening of the interstitial tissue.

5.3.2 Chronic idiopathic polymyositis

The histopathology of chronic polymyositis is summarized in Table 5.3. The main differences between chronic and acute polymyositis are the features of relatively chronic myopathic change (Fig. 5.5), consisting of marked variation in fibre size with hypertrophied fibres, fibre splitting,

Table 5.3 Histological features of chronic idiopathic polymyositis

Myopathic features:
  Marked variation in fibre size
  Hypertrophied fibres
  Central nucleation
  Fibre splitting
  Regenerating and necrotic fibres
  Endomysial and perifascicular fibrosis
Inflammatory cell exudates
Prominent architectural changes in individual fibres, often focally distributed

Neurogenic features:
  Fibre type grouping (usually not prominent)
  Scattered atrophic, pointed, NADH-dark fibres

Fig. 5.5 × 140; NADH. Chronic polymyositis. There is marked variability in fibre size and in the intensity of the enzyme reactivity. Several smaller fibres show increased enzyme reactivity in their rims. Minor 'moth-eaten' architectural changes in the NADH reaction are present. These are non-specific myopathic features. The interfascicular plane is thickened.

central nucleation, regenerating fibres and fibrosis (Fig. 5.6). These changes may resemble those of a limb-girdle dystrophy (Fig. 5.7). However, the diagnosis of chronic polymyositis is suggested by the endomysial inflammatory cell infiltrate (Fig. 5.8) with the myopathic features (Swash and Schwartz, 1977). Further, architectural changes are

Fig. 5.6   × 140; Van Gieson strain. Chronic polymyositis. Sheets of fibrous tissue separate the fascicles and, in some parts of the biopsy, interstitial fibrosis is also prominent. There is a sparse patchy cellular infiltrate mainly in relation to necrotic fibres.

often very prominent in chronic polymyositis and these histological abnormalities are usually focally distributed within the biopsy, whereas in muscular dystrophies the abnormalities are diffusely distributed.

In some biopsies small groups of muscle fibres of the same histochemical type may be noted; in combination with the other histological features this is a characteristic finding. The presence of marked focal inflammatory cell aggregates in a biopsy showing the features of the chronic stage of the disease suggests continuing disease activity, or relapse. In advanced polymyositis, when there has been severe loss of muscle fibres, the biopsy contains islands of abnormal muscle fibres in zones of fatty and fibrous connective tissue. At this late stage of the disease the histological appearances may be non-specific, and similar abnormalities may be found in dystrophies and chronic neurogenic disorders. It is thus important that the biopsy be taken from moderately or mildy affected muscles, rather than from very atrophic muscles.

5.3.3   *Dermatomyositis*

The *adult form* of dermatomyositis is usually idiopathic but it may be associated with malignant neoplasms, especially in people older than 40

Fig. 5.7 × 140; HE. Chronic polymyositis. There is marked variation in fibre size with endomysial fibrosis. Many small fibres are present. The disease is active, as shown by the prominent focal lymphocytic aggregates. The appearance resembles that of limb–girdle muscular dystrophy.

Fig. 5.8 × 140; NADH. Chronic polymyositis. In this section, adjacent to Fig. 5.7, the variable enzyme reactivity of large and small fibres can be seen, showing the diversity of the morphological changes in individual fibres in this disease.

years. In one series, 66% of cases of dermatomyositis in men over this age were associated with cancer but the overall incidence of malignancies in patients with dermatomyositis and polymyositis was only 8% (De Vere and Bradley, 1975). In general, dermatomyositis is a more serious illness than polymyositis, with more severe weakness and greater morbidity and mortality, but dermatomyositis is only a third as common as polymyositis in adults (Rowland *et al.*, 1977).

(a) *Pathology.* The histological features of adult dermatomyositis are indistinguishable from polymyositis without skin involvement. In the *childhood form* of dermatomyositis, vasculitis is a prominent feature of the biopsy, affecting arterioles, capillaries and vessels (Banker and Victor, 1966). Endothelial cell hyperplasia and necrosis leads to occlusion of the capillaries or arterioles and to infarction of groups of muscle fibres or even of part of a fascicle. All the fibres involved in these microinfarcts thus appear to be at the same stage of degeneration or regeneration. Perifascicular atrophy is a marked feature of most biopsies of childhood-onset dermatomyositis (Fig. 5.9), and this is accompanied by a reduction in the number of capillaries in the periphery of these fascicles (Banker, 1975; Carpenter *et al.*, 1976). Muscle capillary endothelial cells contain undulating tubular inclusions and these cells are often surrounded by a reduplicated basal lamina, suggesting that they have previously undergone regeneration (Banker, 1975). Deposition of IgG and complement has been reported in small blood vessels, particularly in veins, in muscle biopsies of childhood-onset dermatomyositis (Whitaker and Engle, 1972), but others have not found this abnormality commonly.

(b) *Skin biopsy.* Skin biopsies may also be helpful in making the diagnosis. The erythematous lesions show changes resembling those found in systemic lupus erythematosus. Epidermal atrophy with oedema of the upper dermis, degeneration of the basal cell layers and a scattered inflammatory cell infiltrate, or features of vasculitis, may be seen. Focal panniculitis of the subcutaneous tissue layers is also a common feature, and calcification may be present.

5.4 Muscle involvement in other autoimmune disorders

Inflammatory myopathy may complicate other autoimmune diseases, and there are some differences in the histological features of the myopathy found in these conditions.

5.4.1 *Polyarteritis nodosa*

In this disease the typical features of acute polymyositis may be found, accompanied by prominent vasculitis, often affecting arterioles, small

Fig. 5.9 Childhood-onset polymyositis (aged 15 years) (a) × 350; HE. Perifascicular atrophy, interfascicular fibrosis and mild architectural changes, especially in the perifascicular region, are the main abnormalities. Small arteries have slightly thickened walls but inflammatory cell exudates are not a feature of the biopsy. (b) × 617; NADH. There are prominent architectural changes, with moth-eaten fibres and perifascicular atrophy.

arteries or veins. The media is most often affected and may become necrotic and eosinophilic. Necrosis extends into the intima leading to thrombus formation within the lumen of the vessel. The internal elastic lamina is almost always involved. Neutrophils and eosinophils are characteristic of the early vascular lesion, but later, lymphocytes, plasma cells and macrophages predominate. At this stage the affected vessels become thickened and nodular. The muscle lesions in polyarteritis nodosa are due to infarction, but haemorrhage may also occur. The lesions vary in age and severity in different parts of the muscle.

Polyarteritis nodosa involves both nerve and muscle (Fig. 5.10). Histological features of denervation, i.e. small, angular, NADH-dark fibres, or of reinnervation, i.e. fibre-type grouping, are characteristic in muscle biopsies in this disorder. At least 30% of patients with polyarteritis nodosa show clinical signs of involvement of muscle; however, muscle biopsy is probably less useful in the diagnosis of this condition than has been suggested in the past (Wallace *et al.*, 1958).

5.4.2   Rheumatoid arthritis

Involvement of muscle is common in rheumatoid arthritis, but active polymyositis is relatively uncommon (Pitkeathley and Coomes, 1966). Type 2 atrophy occurs in muscles relatively immobilized by joint disease, and moth-eaten and whorled fibres may be found. Later, in more advanced cases, atrophy of both fibre types occurs. An inflammatory response in the endomysium and interfascicular tissue, without muscle fibre necrosis or vasculitis, is a common feature of rheumatoid arthritis, occurring in about half the cases (Dubowitz and Brooke, 1973; Haslock *et al.*, 1970).

Disturbances of the innervation of muscle are common in rheumatoid arthritis due to symmetrical polyneuropathy, root lesions or mononeuritis multiplex, especially in patients with rheumatoid vasculitis, and these complications may lead to neurogenic changes in affected muscles, especially in distal muscles.

5.4.3   Systemic lupus erythematosus

Polymyositis is infrequent in systemic lupus, occurring in only 3% of patients in one series (Ester and Christian, 1971). Individual fibres sometimes show vacuoles in association with central nuclei. Although vasculitis is a feature of the disease hyaline thickening, fibrinoid necrosis or thrombotic occlusion of intramuscular blood vessels is uncommon in muscle biopsies (see Fig. 5.11). A sparse lymphocytic endomysial infiltration may be a feature.

Fig. 5.10   × 350; HE. Polyarteritis nodosa. (a) Sural nerve biopsy: this endo-neurial blood vessel, sectioned obliquely, shows lymphocytic infiltration. (b) Cellular infiltration around a thickened small artery in a muscle biopsy.

5.4.4   *Scleroderma (progressive systemic sclerosis)*

Muscular stiffness is common but active polymyositis is a rare complication of this disorder. There are no specific histological features of

Fig. 5.11   × 427; HE. Systemic lupus erythematosus. A dense mononuclear cell infiltrate surrounds a small blood vessel, the wall of which is thickened.

this complication. Muscle biopsies in uncomplicated scleroderma reveal little or no abnormality.

5.4.5   Mixed connective tissue disease

This is a clinical syndrome in which features of various autoimmune disorders coexist. Muscle biopsies often reveal a diffuse, but sparse inflammatory cell exudate, but fibre necrosis or regeneration are relatively uncommon features. In some cases, perivascular inflammatory cell exudates may occur.

5.4.6   Polymyalgia rheumatica

In this disorder muscle stiffness at rest, relieved by activity, is accompanied by fever, malaise and a raised ESR. Most cases occur in women over 55 years of age; there is an association with *temporal arteritis*. The muscle biopsy shows Type 2B fibre atrophy with occasional moth-eaten and whorled fibres. Inflammatory cell infiltrates and increased central nucleation are *not* features of this disorder. These changes resemble those found in mild cases of rheumatoid arthritis.

5.4.7 Eosinophilic fasciitis

This rare disorder resembles idiopathic polyarteritis. The muscle biopsy reveals large numbers of round cells in the fascial planes, with moderate numbers of eosinophils. The muscle shows only mild structural changes (Nassanova *et al.*, 1979) but these may resemble polymyositis in some cases (Stark, 1979).

5.4.8 Infestations of muscle

A variety of parasites have been reported as invading skeletal muscle (Pallis and Lewis, 1981) but infestation of muscle is a rare clinical finding in the United Kingdom, and in other developed countries. Only cysticercosis (*Taenia solium*), trichinosis (*Trichinella spiralis*) and toxocariasis (*Toxocara canis*) are at all likely to be found in muscle biopsies. In trichinosis (Fig. 5.12) the parasite is found inside muscle fibres of either

Fig. 5.12 × 100; paraffin-embedded, HE. Trichinosis of muscle. Two spiral parasites, firmly encased, without reactive cellular response, can be seen (arrows). This represents the chronic, inactive stage of the disease (illustration kindly supplied by Dr Uros Roessman, University Hospitals of Cleveland, Ohio, USA)

histochemical type leading to muscle fibre necrosis, with an intense eosinophilic and macrophage cellular response. In cysticercosis the cysts consist of multiple vesicles surrounded by a mild inflammatory cell exudate in which eosinophils may be prominent. In the late stages these cysts form calcified nodules. Other organs are almost invariably involved. Toxocariasis has been recognized relatively recently as an infestation of children.

5.4.9 Sarcoid myopathy

Although sarcoidosis of muscle may be found coincidentally or on muscle biopsy in about 30% of cases of systemic sarcoidosis, clinically evident sarcoid myopathy is uncommon. The muscle biopsy shows typical sarcoid granulomata, or infiltration with small epithelioid cells (Fig. 5.13). Muscle fibre destruction occurs in the region of the granulomata but isolated degenerating or regenerating muscle fibres are not a feature.

Fig. 5.13 × 140; HE. Sarcoidosis. A granuloma accompanied by an intense lymphocytic cellular infiltrate within the muscle. The multinuclear giant cell was not associated with acid fast bacilli, and the diagnosis of sarcoidosis was confirmed by clinical investigation.

5.4.10 Infections of muscle

Occasionally fungal infection may occur, particularly in patients with overwhelming fungal septicaemia. Bacterial abscesses in muscles develop from contiguous spread from neighbouring infections, e.g. osteomyelitis or cutaneous ulcers, or from haematogenous invasion. Tuberculosis of muscle is very rare. Syphilitic granulomata are also very uncommon.

5.4.11   Myasthenia gravis

Muscle biopsies are not usually performed in the investigation of myasthenia gravis unless there is suspicion of coincidental polymyositis, or a metabolic myopathy, for example hyperthyroid myopathy. Polymyositis and myasthenia gravis may occur in the same patient either at the same time or separately (Johns et al., 1971).

In myasthenia gravis the commonest abnormality is Type 2 fibre atrophy; this was found in about half the biopsies reported by Engel and McFarlin (1966). Type 2 fibre atrophy is not always uniformly distributed, even appearing focally in the biopsy (Dubowitz and Brooke, 1973). Lymphocytic infiltrates, first described by Buzzard (1905) as 'lymphorrhages', consisting of aggregates of lymphocytes situated in the endomysium, unrelated to blood vessels (Russell, 1953) are found in about a quarter of cases biopsied, but are found more commonly at autopsy. Histological features of denervation, consisting of clusters of small, pointed fibres of either histochemical type, or features of reinnervation, e.g. fibre-type grouping, occur in some cases, particularly those in whom the disease has been severe and of considerable duration (Brownell et al., 1972). The motor end-plates show characteristic histological abnormalities both by light and electron microscopy (Coërs et al., 1973), consisting of expanded, proliferated endings, or elongated endings lacking side branches. In addition, there is often increased collateral sprouting at the terminal arborization of the end-plate. Whilst these changes are mainly due to the disease, they may be due, in part to the effects of long-term anticholinesterase therapy (Schwartz et al., 1977).

Myasthenia gravis is a disorder of neuromuscular transmission in which the acetylcholine receptor protein in the motor end-plate is blocked and destroyed by a complement-mediated reaction with a circulating antibody in the IgG compartment. The abnormality is thus postsynaptic and IgG and C3 are deposited at this site (Engel et al., 1977). The postjunctional end-plate membrane is disrupted and the synaptic cleft widened and simplified. This antigen–antibody reaction is accompanied by a local macrophage response and by morphological changes and physiological abnormalities in the motor end-plate which account for the clinical and pathological features of the disease (see Albuquerque et al., 1976 and Swash and Schwartz, 1981 for reviews).

Thymomas are found in 10% of patients with myasthenia gravis; in the remainder the thymus shows hyperplasia, or may be normal.

References

Albuquerque, E. X., Rash, J. E., Mayer, R. F. and Satterfield, R. (1976), Electrophysiological and morphological study of the neuromuscular function in patients with myasthenia gravis. *Expl. Neurol.*, **51**, 536–63.

Banker, B. Q. (1975), Dermatomyositis of childhood: ultrastructural alteration of muscle and intramuscular blood vessels. *J. Neuropath. Expl. Neurol.*, **34**, 46–75.

Banker, B. Q. and Victor, M. (1966), Dermatomyositis (systemic angiopathy) of childhood. *Medicine (Balt.)*, **45**, 261–89.

Brownell, B., Oppenheimer, J. R. and Spalding, J. M. K. (1972), Neurogenic muscle atrophy in myasthenia gravis. *J. Neurol. Neurosurg. Psychiatry*, **34**, 311–22.

Buzzard, E. F. (1905), The clinical history and post mortem examination in five cases of myasthenia gravis. *Brain*, **28**, 438–83.

Carpenter, S., Karpati, G., Rothman, S. and Watters, G. (1976), The childhood type of dermatomyositis. *Neurology (Minneap.)*, **26**, 952–62.

Churg, J. and Strauss, L. (1951), Allergic granulomatosis, allergic angiitis and periarteritis nodosa. *Am. J. Pathol.*, **27**, 277–302.

Coërs, C., Telerman-Toppet, N., Gerard, J-M. (1973), Terminal innervation ratio in neuromuscular disease: disorders of lower motor neuron, peripheral nerve and muscle. *Arch. Neurol.*, **29**, 215–22.

De Vere, R. and Bradley, W. G. (1975), Polymyositis: its presentation, morbidity and mortality. *Brain*, **98**, 637–66.

Dubowitz, V. and Brooke, M. H. (1973), *Muscle Biopsy – a Modern Approach*, W. B. Saunders, London.

Engel, A. G., Lambert, E. H. and Howard, F. M. Jr, (1977), Immune complexes (IgG & C₃) at the motor end plate in myasthenia gravis. *Mayo Clin. Proc.*, **52**, 267–80.

Engel, W. K. and McFarlin, D. E. (1966), Discussion of paper by Fenichel. *Ann. NY Acad. Sci.*, **135**, 68–77.

Ester, D. and Christian, C. L. (1971), The natural history of systemic lupus erythematosus by prospective analysis. *Medicine (Balt.)* **50**, 85–95.

Haslock, D. I., Wright, V. and Harriman, D. G. F. (1970), Neuromuscular disorders in rheumatoid arthritis: a motor point muscle biopsy study. *Q. J. Med.*, **39**, 335–58.

Johns, T. R., Crowley, W. J., Miller, J. Q. and Campa, J. F. (1971), The syndrome of myasthenia and polymyositis, with comments on therapy. *Ann. NY Acad. Sci.*, **183**, 64–71.

Nassanova, V. A., Ivanova, M. M., Akhnazarova, V. D. *et al.* (1979), Eosinophilic fasciitis. *Scand. J. Rheum.*, **8**, 225–33.

Pallis, C. and Lewis, P. D. (1981), Inflammatory myopathies: involvement of human muscle by parasites. In *Disorders of Voluntary Muscle*, 4th edn (ed. J. N. Walton) Churchill Livingstone, Edinburgh, pp. 569–84.

Pitkeathley, D. A. and Coomes, E. N. (1966), Polymyositis in rheumatoid arthritis. *Ann. Rheum. Dis.*, **25**, 127–32.

Rowland, L. P., Clarke, C. and Clark, M. (1977), Therapy for dermatomyositis

94   Biopsy Pathology of Muscle

and polymyositis. In *Advances in neurology*, Vol. 17, (eds R. C. Griggs and R. T. Moxley III), Ravel Press, New York.

Russell, D. S. (1953), Histological changes in the striped muscles in myasthenia gravis. *J. Pathol.*, **65**, 279–89.

Schwartz, M. S., Sargeant, M. K. and Swash, M. (1977), Neostigmine-induced end plate proliferation in the rat. *Neurology (Minneap.)*, **27**, 289–93.

Stark, R. J. (1979), Eosinophilic polymyositis. *Arch. Neurol.*, **36**, 721–2.

Swash, M. and Schwartz, M. S. (1977), Implications of longitudinal muscle fibre splitting in neurogenic and myopathic disorders. *J. Neurol. Neurosurg. Psychiatry*, **40**, 1152–9.

Swash, M. and Schwartz, M. S. (1981), *Neuromuscular Diseases: A Practical Approach to Diagnosis and Management*, Springer-Verlag, Berlin, Heidelberg, New York.

Swash, M., Schwartz, M. S. and Sargeant, M. K. (1978), Pathogenesis of longitudinal splitting of muscle fibres in neurogenic disorders and in polymyositis. *Neuropathol. Appl. Neurobiol.*, **4**, 99–115.

Wallace, S. L., Lattis, R. and Ragan, C. (1958), Diagnostic significance of the muscle biopsy. *Am. J. Med.*, **25**, 600–10.

Whitaker, J. N. (1982), Inflammatory myopathy: a review of etiologic and pathogenic features. *Muscle Nerve*, **5**, 573–97.

Whitaker, J. N. and Engel W. K. (1972), Vascular deposits of immunoglobulin and complement in idiopathic inflammatory myopathy. *New Eng. J. Med.*, **286**, 333–8.

6 Muscular dystrophies

The muscular dystrophies are relatively uncommon inherited disorders of muscle. They are characterized by a progressive course and by degenerative changes in skeletal muscle fibres. Most begin in childhood but in others the disease is not recognized until adult life. Classification depends on clinical, genetic and histological criteria (Table 6.1). The childhood myopathies are, by convention, classified separately since these disorders are only very slowly progressive and they show only mild myopathic changes in the muscle, although there may be particular features in certain of these disorders.

Table 6.1 Classification of muscular dystrophies

X-linked muscular dystrophies
Duchenne muscular dystrophy
Becker muscular dystrophy
Other X-linked, less severe muscular dystrophies
Scapulo-peroneal muscular dystrophy
Limb girdle muscular dystrophy
Facio-scapulo-humeral muscular dystrophy
Myotonic dystrophy and other myotonic syndromes
Ocular myopathies
Oculo-pharyngeal dystrophy

6.1 Duchenne muscular dystrophy

This disorder is the commonest form of muscular dystrophy. It is inherited as an X-linked recessive disorder, so that it affects boys only, although cases of affected girls with Turner's syndrome (XO) have been reported. The trait is carried on the short arm of the X chromosome. In affected families in which the mother is known to be a carrier of the gene, half the boys will be affected, and half the girls will be carriers. However, it has been estimated that as many as a third of affected boys represent new mutations and in these cases none of the

95

relatives will be carriers. Female carriers may show minor abnormalities, such as hypertrophied calf muscles, slight proximal muscle weakness and, more frequently, a raised CK, and these features are often used to establish the carrier state in genetic counselling (see Harper, 1982).

Affected boys always develop the full clinical syndrome. Weakness of girdle muscles, especially pelvic muscles, is apparent before the age of 4 years. Hypertrophy of muscles, especially calves, deltoids and serratus anterior, is an important diagnostic feature. Slight intellectual impairment and an abnormal ECG are often found. The child never runs, and walking is abnormal, with a characteristic waddling, broad-based gait and lordotic posture. Motor milestones are delayed. Most patients lose the ability to walk by the age of 11 years and about 75% die before the age of 21 years. Survival beyond 30 years is unusual (Walton and Gardner-Medwin, 1981).

The CK is greatly raised in all cases, especially in the early stages of the disorder when it may be 20 or more times normal. In female carriers the CK is only slightly raised; in some it may be normal.

6.1.1   Muscle pathology

The changes in muscle biopsies vary according to the stage of the disease (Table 6.2).

The most characteristic histological feature of Duchenne dystrophy is the presence of hyaline fibres (Fig. 6.1); these are especially prominent in

Table 6.2 Sequence of muscle biopsy changes in Duchenne dystrophy

	Early 1–5 years ambulant	Moderately advanced 6–10 years marked weakness	Late 10 years or older chairbound
Hyalinized fibres	────────────	────────────	
Fibre necrosis	────────────	────────────	------------
Phagocytosis	────────────	────────────	------------
Fibrosis	------------	────────────	────────────
Rounded fibres	------------	────────────	────────────
Regenerating fibres	────────────	────────────	
Central nucleation		────────────	────────────
Fibre splitting		────────────	────────────
Fibre hypertrophy		────────────	────────────
Fat replacement	------------	------------	────────────
Poor fibre-type differentiation	────────────	────────────	────────────

Fig. 6.1 Duchenne muscular dystrophy, × 180; HE. In this paraffin-embedded section a muscle spindle, sectioned through its nuclear bag region, is prominent; its periaxial space is enlarged and contains unusually prominent inner capsular connective tissue. There are fewer than the normal 6–14 intrafusal muscle fibres. In the muscle itself hyaline fibres, which appear dark, rounded and large, are prominent. There is increased endomysial fibrosis.

the early stages of the disease. They are large rounded fibres which appear homogeneous and vitreous in HE stains. In longitudinal sections the cross-striations are lost. Hyaline fibres stain slightly darker than other fibres, including HE (Fig. 6.7), Gomori and NADH techniques, (Fig. 6.2) and they are a particular feature of the early stage of the disease. Hyaline fibres probably result from hypercontraction of parts of muscle fibres due to uncontrolled entry of calcium into these fibres through defects in the plasma membrane. Calcium is concentrated at the edges of these fibres (Fig. 6.3), and this can be demonstrated histologically (Bodensteiner and Engel, 1978). Hyaline change may thus represent the first stage in necrosis of muscle fibres in this disease (Cullen and Fulthorpe, 1975). Walton (1973) noted that in serial sections, adjacent parts of affected fibres are often necrotic and undergoing phagocytosis. Hyaline fibres are not specific for Duchenne dystrophy since they also occur, although in fewer numbers, in other X-linked dystrophies and, rarely, in limb–girdle dystrophy.

Fig. 6.2 Duchenne muscular dystrophy. × 140; NADH. The fascicles are separated by thickened unstained interfascicular connective tissue. The muscle fibres vary in size and several show zones of increased reactivity. The differentiation fibre types is less developed than in normal muscle.

Fig. 6.3 Duchenne muscular dystrophy, × 350; Alizarin red. Three fibres stain intensely, indicating increased calcium content. There are hyaline fibres. Some stain has precipitated on the surface of the section producing areas of dark artefact.

Necrotic fibres undergoing phagocytosis are common in the early and moderately advanced stages of the disease. These are often surrounded by small round cells and macrophages. Clusters of small basophilic regenerating fibres are usually a prominent feature (Fig. 6.4), especially in the earlier stages of the disease. They may be found at any site within a fascicle and they are often associated with an inflammatory cell infiltrate in the endomysium. These fibres usually contain acid phosphatase (Fig. 6.5) as well as sarcoplasmic RNA (Neerunjun and Dubowitz, 1977). The sarcoplasm of these fibres is vesicular and their nuclei contain a dispersed chromatin pattern.

In the middle stages of the disease the muscle fibres appear rounded and show increased variability in size (Fig. 6.6). There is marked interfascicular and endomysial fibrosis even in the early stages when the fascicular pattern is preserved (Fig. 6.7), and the majority of muscle fibres are relatively undamaged. In enzyme histochemical stains fibre-type differentiation is poorly developed in the ATPase preparations so that it may be difficult to distinguish the Type 1 and Type 2 fibres (Fig. 6.6). When fibre types can be differentiated there is a deficiency of Type 2B fibres but an increased number of Type 2C fibres in most cases. Fibre-type differentiation in the NADH, SDH, glycogen and phosphorylase reactions appear normal, but morphological changes in individual fibres may be demonstrated with these techniques. Both fibre types appear equally involved in degenerative and regenerative changes (Engel, 1977).

Splitting of muscle fibres may be a prominent feature at a stage of the disease at which the child is still mobile, usually between the ages of 5 and 7 years (Bell and Conen, 1968), but it becomes less prominent later. Muscle fibre hypertrophy is not usually prominent, although the hyaline fibres themselves are larger than the surrounding fibres. The distribution of blood vessels and capillaries in relation to individual muscle fibres is normal. Muscle spindles show thickening of their capsule and enlargement of their periaxial spaces (Fig. 6.1) but are usually relatively well-preserved until the most advanced stage of the disorder (Swash and Fox, 1976). Intramuscular nerve bundles appear normal, even when the muscle is largely destroyed; methylene blue impregnations have shown enlargement of the innervational area of motor end-plates but no collateral sprouting (Coërs and Tellerman-Toppet, 1977).

Electron microscopy is not helpful in diagnosis, but it has been used to demonstrate discontinuities in the plasma membrane of muscle fibres; and it has been suggested that this may be part of an underlying membrane disorder leading to the histological features of the disease (Carpenter and Karpati, 1979; Mokri and Engel, 1975; Rowland, 1980).

Fig. 6.4 Duchenne muscular dystrophy. × 350; HE. Zones of clustered regenerating fibres (arrows), of varying size and staining characteristics. Some contain central or plump sarcolemmal nuclei, and the fibres vary greatly in size. Some nearby rounded fibres show ice-crystal artefact.

Fig. 6.5 Duchenne muscular dystrophy. × 350; Acid phosphatase. Several small fibres or fibre fragments, associated with necrosis and subsequent regeneration, show a positive reaction (arrow). This is usually associated with lysosomal activity.

Fig. 6.6 Duchenne muscular dystrophy. × 140; ATPase, pH 4.6. Poor fibre-type differentiation. Note the rounded fibres and their wide separation from each other.

Fig. 6.7 Duchenne muscular dystrophy. × 140; HE. The muscle fibres are all unusually rounded and there are many darkly staining (eosinophilic) hyaline fibres. There is endomysial and interfascicular fibrosis. Adipose tissue is prominent. A nerve bundle appears normal. Several clusters of small atrophic regenerating fibres are present.

6.1.2   Changes in the fetus

Increased variation in muscle fibre diameter, an increase in the amount of connective tissue and hyalinized fibres have been described in fetuses of 18–20 weeks gestation presumed, on the basis of a family history of the disease and raised placental blood CK levels, to have muscular dystrophy (Emery and Burt, 1980; Mahoney et al., 1977). The significance of these changes in the diagnosis of the disease in neonates, or in stillborn infants, is uncertain.

6.1.3   Changes in carriers

Muscle biopsy has been used as part of the investigation of a suspected carrier, but it is now rarely used, since a raised blood CK level is a more reliable indicator of carrier status. Some carriers show hypertrophy of muscles and muscle biopsy may show muscle fibre hypertrophy in these cases. Other changes include increased central nucleation, increased variability in fibre size, fibre splitting and occasional basophilic fibres (Dubowitz and Brooke, 1973). However, these changes, when they occur, are usually slight; their absence does not exclude the carrier state. They are probably more common in young than in older carrier females.

6.2   Becker muscular dystrophy

This disorder is of later onset and slower progression than Duchenne dystrophy so that survival into adult life is usual and affected men may remain relatively mobile until the 4th decade. Although Becker muscular dystrophy is inherited as an X-linked disorder (Becker and Kiener, 1955) it is almost certainly genetically distinct from Duchenne disease. The CK is raised to a similar degree to that found in Duchenne muscular dystrophy.

6.2.1   Muscle pathology

The muscle biopsy resembles that of Duchenne muscular dystrophy in some respects, particularly in the presence of rounded fibres, central nucleation, split fibres and endomysial fibrosis, but there are several points of difference. Hyaline fibres are relatively uncommon, fibre-type differentiation is not impaired, and clusters of small, angular NADH-dark fibres are often a feature (Bradley et al., 1978). The latter may suggest a neurogenic process but the widespread dystrophic change is distinctive, and diagnostic of the disorder (Fig. 6.8).

Fig. 6.8 Becker muscular dystrophy, × 180; HE. The abnormality in many respects resembles that of Duchenne muscular dystrophy, with marked regenerative fibre clusters.

6.3   Other X-linked dystrophies

Several mild forms of X-linked muscular dystrophy have been described. Clinically, these cases resemble Becker's dystrophy, although they may begin even later, and follow a milder course. Only few such families have been described (Mabry *et al.*, 1965; Ringel *et al.*, 1977). The muscle biopsy shows features resembling Duchenne and Becker type muscular dystrophies in that hyaline fibres are present and there is variability in fibre size, with central nucleation and some increase in endomysial fibrous tissue. However, the histological abnormality is relatively less severe. An X-linked form of scapulo-peroneal muscular dystrophy has also been reported; its histological features resemble those of limb-girdle muscular dystrophy (see Swash *et al.*, 1983, for review).

6.4   Limb–girdle muscular dystrophy

The limb–girdle dystrophy syndrome (Walton and Nattrass, 1954) consists of a wide spectrum of progressive muscular disorders with a variable pattern of inheritance, although an autosomal recessive trait is common. Muscular weakness usually becomes apparent in the 2nd or 3rd decade and progresses slowly so that disability becomes severe only 20 years or more after the onset of the disorder. The CK level is raised, but not to the degree found in Duchenne dystrophy. Many cases formerly classified as limb–girdle muscular dystrophy have been found on reinvestigation, using modern enzyme histochemical muscle biopsy techniques, to have a neurogenic basis for their muscular weakness, usually spinal muscular atrophy of the Kugelberg–Welander type.

6.4.1 Muscle Pathology

The muscle biopsy shows typical myopathic features (Fig. 6.9). In some biopsies muscle fibre hypertrophy is prominent, with muscle fibres up to 200 μm in transverse diameter. Central nucleation and fibre splitting may also be prominent. Various other morphological changes including whorled fibres (Fig. 6.10) sarcoplasmic masses, vacuolated fibres and peripheral accumulations of NADH-dark material may occur. Scattered

Fig. 6.9 Limb-girdle dystrophy, × 427; HE. There is very marked fibre hypertrophy. One fibre (arrow) is undergoing splitting – another shows an artefactual split induced during section processing.

Fig. 6.10 Limb–girdle dystrophy, × 350; NADH. Fibre hypertrophy is prominent. A whorled fibre, in which abnormalities of myofilament orientation and distribution are accompanied by similar changes in mitochondrial distribution, is a very striking abnormality.

necrotic and regenerating fibres are found but these are not prominent features of this slowly progressive disorder. Endomysial and interfascicular fibrosis and fat replacement occur in the advanced stages of the disorder (Fig. 6.11), when there has been extensive loss of muscle fibres. Small rounded atrophic fibres may persist in areas of fibrous tissue, amongst scattered or isolated hypertrophied fibres. Sparse lymphocytic infiltration, often also containing macrophages, may be found in association with necrotic or regenerating fibres. Generally proximal leg muscles show more abnormality than proximal arm muscles and quadriceps biopsies are therefore more likely to show typical abnormalities than deltoid biopsies. Sometimes the vastus internus is more atrophic than the lateral part of the quadriceps.

In some cases more specific histological abnormalities have been recognized. For example, the presence of extensively vacuolated Type 1 fibres, with dense accumulation of glycogen and acid phosphatase-positive material are features associated with acid maltase deficiency (Type II glycogenosis), a disorder which may present in adult life as a slowly progressive myopathy resembling the syndrome of limb–girdle dystrophy (Engel, 1970; Hudgson *et al.*, 1968). Although there are variations in the pathological features of individual cases of limb–girdle

Fig. 6.11 Limb–girdle dystrophy. × 140 (a) HE. There is marked fibre
hypertrophy, but also fibre atrophy, rounded fibres, fibre splitting, fibrosis, fat
replacement, and increased central nucleation. (b) ATPase, pH 4.3. There is
marked variation in fibre size, with increased numbers of Type 2C fibres (the
fibres with an intermediate reaction between the dark Type 1 and pale Type 2A
and Type 2B fibres). Fibre splitting is occurring in several fibres.

dystrophy no specific features have been recognized and definitive subclassification of this syndrome has not yet been accomplished.

An important disorder to be considered in the differential diagnosis of limb–girdle muscular dystrophy is low-grade or chronic polymyositis. This disorder can usually be readily differentiated by muscle biopsy, particularly by the presence of inflammatory cell infiltrates, when this occurs. Polymyositis is also characterized by active necrosis and regeneration, and by prominent architectural changes in individual fibres. Polymyositis, in addition, often shows a rather focal distribution of abnormality.

6.5 Facio-scapulo-humeral muscular dystrophy

This rare disorder is inherited as an autosomal dominant trait. Weakness usually involves face and shoulder girdle musculature, particularly biceps brachii and periscapular muscles. Involvement of the hip occurs later, particularly affecting anterior tibial muscles. Facial weakness may be a prominent presenting feature in childhood with little other abnormality until middle age but a severe childhood onset form of the disease has also been described.

6.5.1 Muscle Biopsy

In many patients the biopsy may be virtually normal, with occasional small round fibres as the only abnormal feature (Fig. 6.12). Since the shoulder girdle muscles are preferentially affected abnormalities are more prominent in upper than in lower limb muscles and biopsies should therefore always be taken from biceps brachii or deltoid muscles. Even in weak muscles abnormalities are not as striking as in other muscular dystrophies. Some fibres, especially Type 1 fibres, show whorled or moth-eaten changes (Dubowitz and Brooke, 1973) and small angular fibres, strongly reactive in oxidative enzyme reactions (e.g. NADH) are often found. The latter do not occur in groups as in neurogenic disorders. Hypertrophic fibres are also common but central nucleation and fibre splitting are infrequent and fibrosis is rare.

In some cases an inflammatory cell reaction may be a striking feature, and it may appear nodular (Munsat et al., 1972). In the more rapidly progressive cases this inflammatory change is sometimes associated with necrotic fibres but necrotic and regenerating fibres are uncommon in most cases of facio-scapulo-humeral dystrophy and the significance of this inflammatory cell reaction is unknown. Munsat et al. (1972) and Munsat and Bradley (1977) considered that some of these patients might be suffering from polymyositis, but there is no response to steroid

Fig. 6.12 Facio-scapulo-humeral dystrophy. × 140; HE. There are only mild abnormalities consisting of a few small fibres and increased perimysial and endomysial fibrous connective tissue. Nerve fibres are prominent. Fibre necrosis and other changes are not a feature.

treatment in this form of muscular dystrophy. The differential diagnosis can be made by the family history, and by the presence of hypertrophied fibres, which are uncommon in polymyositis, even in the chronic phase.

Van Wijngaarden and Bethlem (1973) in a review of patients with weakness in a facio-scapulo-humeral distribution, mostly of sporadic occurrence, noted that a wide variety of neuromuscular disorders might be responsible, including polymyositis, myasthenia gravis, congenital myopathies and mitochondrial myopathies, in addition to facio-scapulo-humeral dystrophy.

6.6 Myotonic dystrophy

Myotonic dystrophy is a dominantly inherited disorder, which shows marked variability in severity within individual pedigrees. Since mild forms of the disease are common, the diagnosis is often missed. On the other hand, the typical clinical features are well known and in patients with the fully developed disorder muscle biopsy is usually not required for diagnosis. Furthermore, muscle biopsy is not useful in the diagnosis of patients in whom there is clinical uncertainty. Electromyography is far more useful, since it allows detection of the characteristic myotonia and provides evidence for a myopathy.

The most important clinical features are myotonia, weakness more marked in distal than in proximal muscles, causing weakness of the hands, and foot drop. The tendon reflexes are often absent. Systemic involvement is usual and includes cataract, endocrine disturbances, e.g. diabetes mellitus, testicular atrophy and infertility, dysphagia from involvement of the smooth muscle of the oesophagus, respiratory distress, and abnormalities of cardiac conduction including heart block. Mental abnormalities are frequent. Among affected adults men and women are equally affected, but the children of mothers with the disease may show a severe abnormality, with failure to thrive, respiratory distress, floppiness and weakness, marked facial weakness and mental retardation. The children of fathers with the disease are much less likely to develop this syndrome of *congenital myotonic dystrophy*.

6.6.1   Muscle biopsy

In the adult form of myotonic dystrophy the major abnormality is central nucleation (Fig. 6.13); frequently chains of central nuclei or multiple internal nuclei may be found (Figs. 6.13 and 6.14). This is best seen in longitudinal sections. Very small fibres containing aggregations of dense nuclei are common and there is increased variability in fibre size (Fig.

Fig. 6.13 Myotonic dystrophy. × 140; HE. Fibre hypertrophy with increased central nucleation are the main features (mean fibre diameter 81 µm; approximately 3 central nuclei per muscle fibre – the normal is <0.04 representing 4% fibres with central nuclei).

Fig. 6.14   Myotonic dystrophy. × 350; HE. This longitudinal section shows the tendency for internal nuclei to be arranged in chains (usually not a striking phenomenon), and the characteristic, slightly basophilic, tiny atrophic fibres, containing large, dark nuclei. The latter fibres resemble those found in chronic denervation atrophy. The wavy appearance is an artefact of section preparation.

6.15), with selective atrophy of Type 1 fibres, and hypertrophy of Type 2 fibres. Fibre splitting is sometimes prominent and ring fibres, in which displaced myofibrils appear to encircle the fibre beneath the plasma membrane in transverse sections, are an especially characteristic, but non-specific feature (Fig. 6.16). Sarcoplasmic masses, consisting of zones of clear or granular sarcoplasm occur at the periphery of muscle fibres, both in adult and childhood onset cases.

The most characteristic abnormality in the muscle biopsy in myotonic dystrophy is found in the muscle spindles (Daniel and Strich, 1964). This abnormality is likely to be detected only in biopsies taken from distal muscles, e.g. flexor muscles of the forearm, since the disease affects distal muscles more than proximal muscles, and spindles are found in greater number in distal than in proximal muscles. The change consists of fragmentation of the intrafusal muscle fibres, so that there appears to be a marked increase in the number of intrafusal muscle fibres in affected spindles (Fig. 6.17). Thickening and fibrosis of the spindle capsule are also features of the abnormality. Normal spindles contain less than 14 intrafusal fibres but in myotonic dystrophy there may be as many as 100 separate tiny fragments in a single spindle in transverse section (Swash, 1972). Ultrastructural studies show a marked variation in the appearance

Fig. 6.15 Myotonic dystrophy. × 350; HE. The smaller fibres are more darkly stained (eosinophilic). These are atrophic Type 2 fibres. Central nucleation is not always a feature of the disease.

of individual fibre fragments (Swash and Fox, 1975a; b), which is well demonstrated in serial sections. Not all the muscle spindles in a given muscle are abnormal, but the innervation of these abnormal spindles is disturbed, with marked proliferation of sensory and motor axons (Swash, 1972).

The motor innervation of extrafusal muscle fibres is also abnormal. There is expansion of the terminal arborization and prominent axonal branching leading to innervation of several adjacent muscle fibres by these branches (Coërs *et al.*, 1973).

In congenital myotonic dystrophy the biopsy is less abnormal. Central nucleation and fibre hypertrophy occur and sarcoplasmic masses may sometimes be prominent, but ring fibres are rarely a feature.

6.6.2   *Other myotonic syndromes*

There are two forms of myotonia congenita, a familial disorder characterized by myotonia without dystrophic features or signs of multisystem involvement. Muscle hypertrophy occurs in both the dominantly inherited form (Thomsen's disease) and in the recessive form (Becker's variant) but in the latter, mild distal atrophy and weakness may develop in the course of the disease. Paramyotonia congenita, in which

Fig. 6.17 Myotonic dystrophy. × 350; Toluidine blue, plastic section. The intrafusal muscle fibres are fragmented, either because of multiple splitting, or from abortive regenerative activity. The spindle capsule is thickened.

myotonia is markedly enhanced by cold, is also inherited as a dominant trait without systemic involvement.

The muscle biopsy in these conditions shows fibre hypertrophy, and there may be some scattered atrophic fibres (Fig. 6.18). Necrotic fibres are uncommon, and only a few fibres show central nucleation. Type 2B fibres may be absent (Crews *et al.*, 1976). Muscle spindles are normal in this condition (Swash and Schwartz, 1983).

6.7 Ocular myopathies and oculo-pharyngeal dystrophy

Ptosis and chronic progressive external ophthalmoplegia, due to muscular rather than cranial nerve or central nervous system disease, may occur alone or in association with weakness of pharyngeal muscles. In many patients there is slight associated weakness of proximal muscles, especially of the upper limbs. In the oculo-cranio-somatic syndrome

Fig. 6.16 Myotonic dystrophy. × 140; (a) ATPase, pH 9.5. Type 2 atrophy, with multiple central nucleation in fibres of both histochemical types, can be a distinctive feature of the disease. (b) Myotonic dystrophy. EM × 15 000. A peripheral myofibril is displaced into a 'ring' position, and there is a peripheral sarcoplasmic mass.

Fig. 6.18   Myotonia congenita. × 152; ATPase, pH 4.6. Scattered atrophic fibres (<30 μm) without hypertrophic fibres. Two fibres are vacuolated, or show core formation.

systemic involvement, including cerebellar ataxia, deafness, retinitis pigmentosa, heart block and cortico-spinal signs, may occur; in this syndrome muscle biopsy may reveal abnormal mitochondria, a feature related to the mitochondrial myopathies (Chapter 8). Central core disease, and related syndromes may also cause mild proximal weakness with involvement of the external ocular muscles (Chapter 7).

6.7.1   Muscle biopsy

Limb muscle biopsies in oculo-pharyngeal dystrophy show minor abnormalities including variability in fibre size with some hypertrophied fibres, scattered small angular fibres, darkly reactive in NADH preparations, some whorled or moth-eaten fibres but no necrotic or degenerating fibres. Ultrastructural studies have revealed filamentous inclusions in muscle fibre nuclei in this condition (Tomé and Fardeau, 1980). Limb muscle biopsies in patients with ocular myopathy alone may show ragged-red fibres with little other abnormality.

References

Bell, C. D. and Conen, P. E. (1968), Histopathological changes in Duchenne muscular dystrophy. *J. Neurol. Sci.*, **7**, 529–44.

Becker, P. E. and Kiener, F. (1955), Eine neue X chromosale Muskel dystrophie. *Arch. Psychiat. Nervenkr.*, **193**, 427–48.

Bodensteiner, J. B. and Engel, A. G. (1978), Intracellular calcium accumulation in Duchenne dystrophy and other myopathies: a study of 567,000 muscle fibres in 114 biopsies. *Neurology (NY)*, **28**, 439–46.

Bradley, W. G., Jones, M. Z., Mussini, J. M. and Fawcett, P. R. W. (1978), Becker-type muscular dystrophy. *Muscle Nerve*, **1**, 111–32.

Carpenter, S. and Karpati, G. (1979), Duchenne muscular dystrophy: plasma membrane loss initiated muscle cell necrosis unless it is repaired. *Brain*, **102**, 147–61.

Coërs, C. and Tellerman-Toppet, N. (1977), Morphological changes of motor units in Duchenne's muscular dystrophy. *Arch. Neurol.*, **34**, 396–402.

Coërs, C., Tellerman-Toppet, N. and Gerard, J.-M. (1973), Terminal innervation ratio in neuromuscular disease: disorders of lower motor neuron, peripheral nerve and muscle. *Arch. Neurol.*, **29**, 215–22.

Crews, J., Kaiser, K. K. and Brooke, M. H. (1976), Muscle pathology of myotonia congenita. *J. Neurol. Sci.*, **28**, 449–57.

Cullen, M. J. and Fulthorpe, J. J. (1975), Stages in fibre breakdown in Duchenne muscular dystrophy. An electromicroscopic study. *J. Neurol. Sci.*, **24**, 179–200.

Daniel, P. M. and Strich, S. J. (1964), Abnormalities in the muscle spindles in dystrophia myotonica. *Neurology (Minneap.)*, **14**, 310–16.

Dubowitz, V. and Brooke, M. H. (1973), *Muscle Biopsy – A Modern Approach*, W. B. Saunders, London.

Emery, A. E. H. and Burt, D. E. (1980), Intracellular calcium and pathogenesis and antenatal diagnosis of Duchenne muscular dystrophy. *Br. Med. J.*, **280**, 355–7.

Engel, A. G. (1970), Acid maltase deficiency in adults. *Brain*, **93**, 599–606.

Engel, W. K. (1977), Integrative histochemical approach to the defect in muscular dystrophy. In *Pathogenesis of Human Muscular Dystrophies* (ed. L. P. Rowland), Excerpta Medica, Amsterdam, pp. 277–309.

Harper, P. S. (1982), Carrier detection in Duchenne muscular dystrophy: a critical assessment. In *Disorders of the Motor Unit* (ed. D. L. Schotland) Wiley Medical, New York, ch. 63, pp. 821–46, 847–60.

Hudgson, P., Gardner-Medwin, D., Worsfold, M. *et al.* (1968), Adult myopathy from glycogen storage disease due to acid maltase deficiency. *Brain*, **91**, 435–62.

Mabry, C. C., Rockel, I. E., Morwick, R. L. and Robertson, D. (1965), X linked pseudo hypertrophic muscular dystrophy with a late onset and slow progression. *New Engl. J. Med.*, **273**, 1062–70.

Mahoney, M. J., Haseltine, F. P. and Hobbins, J. C. (1977), Prenatal diagnosis of Duchenne muscular dystrophy. *New Engl. J. Med.*, **297**, 968–73.

Mokri, B. and Engel, A. G. (1975), Duchenne dystrophy: electron microscopic findings pointing to a basic or early abnormality in the plasma membrane of the muscle fibre. *Neurology* (Minneap.), **25**, 1111–20.

Munsat, T. L. and Bradley, W. G. (1977), Serum creatine phosphokinase levels and prednisone-treated muscle weakness. *Neurology (Minneap.)*, **27**, 96–7.

Munsat, T. L., Piper, O., Canulla, P. and Mednik, J. (1972), Inflammatory myopathy with facio-scapulo-humeral distribution. *Neurology (Minneap.)*, **22**, 335–47.

Neerunjun, S. J. S. and Dubowitz, V. (1977), Concomitance of basophilia, ribonucleic acid and acid phosphatase activity in regenerating muscle fibres. *J. Neurol. Sci.*, **33**, 95–109.

Ringel, S. P., Carroll, J. E. and Schold, S. C. (1977), The spectrum of mild X-linked recessive muscular dystrophy. *Arch. Neurol.*, **34**, 408–16.

Rowland, L. P. (1980), Biochemistry of muscle membranes in Duchenne muscular dystrophy. *Muscle Nerve*, **3**, 3–20.

Swash, M. (1972), The morphology and innervation of the muscle spindle in dystrophia myotonica. *Brain*, **95**, 357–68.

Swash, M. and Fox, K. P. (1975a), Abnormal intrafusal muscle fibres in myotonic dystrophy: a study using serial sections. *J. Neurol. Neurosurg. Psychiatry*, **38**, 91–9.

Swash, M. and Fox, K. P. (1975b), The fine structure of the spindle abnormality in myotonic dystrophy. *Neuropath. Appl. Neurobiol.*, **1**, 171–87.

Swash, M. and Fox, K. P. (1976), The pathology of the muscle spindle in Duchenne muscular dystrophy. *J. Neurol. Sci.*, **29**, 17–32.

Swash, M. and Schwartz, M. S. (1983), Normal muscle spindle morphology in myotonia congenita. *Clin. Neuropathol.*, **2**, 75–8.

Swash, M. Schwartz, M. S., Carter, N. D. *et al.* (1983), Benign X-linked myopathy with acanthocytes (McLeod syndrome) – its relationship to X-linked muscular dystrophy. *Brain*, **106**, 717–34.

Tomé, F. and Fardeau, M. (1980), Nuclear inclusions in oculopharyngeal dystrophy. *Acta Neuropathol. (Berlin)*, **49**, 85–7.

van Wijngaarden, G. K. and Bethlem, J. (1973), The facio-scapulo-humeral syndrome. In *Clinical Studies in Myology* (ed. B. A. Kakulas), Exerpta Medica, Amsterdam, pp. 498–501.

Walton, J. N. (1973), Progressive muscular dystrophy: structural alteration in various stages and in carriers of muscular dystrophy. In *The Striated Muscle* (ed. C. M. Pearson), Williams and Wilkins, Baltimore, pp. 263–91.

Walton, J. N. and Gardner-Medwin, D. (1981), Progressive muscular dystrophy and the myotonic disorders. In *Disorders of Voluntary Muscle*, 4th edn (ed. J. N. Walton), Churchill Livingstone, Edinburgh, pp. 481–524.

Walton, J. N. and Nattrass, F. T. (1954), On the classification, natural history and treatment of the myopathies. *Brain*, **77**, 169–231.

7 'Benign' myopathies of childhood

The term 'benign myopathies of childhood' is used to describe a group of disorders characterized clinically by the 'floppy infant syndrome'. They are sometimes referred to as *congenital myopathies*, although in some instances they may not cause symptoms until later in childhood or even until adult life. These disorders usually have a genetic basis, although this may not be apparent. In most patients weakness is mild or moderate, and marked wasting is unusual. These disorders are usually only slowly progressive and, in some, improvement may occur with increasing maturity (Dubowitz, 1978; 1980). There are many causes of the floppy infant syndrome (Table 7.1) but many of these are best reclassified according to their underlying cause, e.g. as metabolic myopathies, leaving a group of ill-understood, relatively benign myopathies of childhood onset characterized principally by the changes found in the muscle biopsy (Table 7.2).

Hypotonia occurring in children of normal intelligence, with retained tendon reflexes and normal active movements of the limbs, is unlikely to have a serious or progressive underlying cause. If improvement occurs in a few months and the CK is normal, no further investigation is required. Lundberg (1979) found that only 4% of a group of such floppy babies had an underlying neuromuscular disorder. In a series of infants with hypotonia, associated with other features of neurological disorder, Paine (1963) found that 73% had central nervous system disease, 16% were categorized as benign congenital myopathy and 3% had a myopathy or spinal muscular atrophy, respectively. Myopathies of infancy and childhood are thus uncommon disorders.

7.1 Nemaline myopathy

This is probably the commonest of the congenital myopathies presenting in childhood. The disease may present in infancy or in childhood; the disorder varies greatly from case to case but is generally most severe in

117

Table 7.1 Causes of floppy infant syndrome

Central nervous system disease
  Cerebral palsy
  Mental retardation
  Cerebellar disease
  Spinal cord injury

Neurogenic disorders
  Type 1 spinal muscular atrophy (Werdnig–Hoffmann)
  Poliomyelitis
  Peripheral neuropathy

Infantile myasthenia gravis

Myopathies
  Congenital muscular dystrophy
  Myopathies with structural changes in the muscle biopsy (see Table 7.2)
  Metabolic myopathies of childhood (see Chapter 8)
  Myotonic dystrophy

Others (usually without weakness)
  Benign congenital hypotonia
  Ehlers–Danlos and related syndromes
  Prader–Willi syndrome
  Reversible metabolic disorders, e.g. hypoglycaemia
  Hypothyroidism and other endocrine disorders

Table 7.2 *'Benign' myopathies of childhood* (childhood-onset myopathies with slow progression and structural changes in the muscle biopsy)

Nemaline myopathy
  Central core and multicore (minicore) disease
  Myotubular (centronuclear) myopathy
  Congenital fibre type disproportion
  Myopathy with tubular aggregates
  Failure of fibre type differentiation

Others
  Myopathy with finger-print inclusions
  Zebra body myopathy
  Megaconial and pleoconial myopathies?
  Congenital muscular dystrophy

cases of infantile onset. In the latter, respiratory problems may be a feature. The tendon reflexes are usually absent and skeletal abnormalities, e.g. kyphoscoliosis and pes cavus, may be present. Nemaline myopathy is usually an autosomal recessive disorder but dominant cases are known.

7.1.1   Muscle biopsy

The cardinal feature is the presence of rod-like inclusions (Fig. 7.1), which appear red in the Gomori trichrome preparation, faintly basophilic in HE stains and blue in PTAH preparations. In HE stains they are best seen by phase microscopy (Hudgson *et al.*, 1967). The rod bodies are usually mainly subsarcolemmal in location. They vary in length from 1–5 μm and in diameter from 0.2–2.0 μm (Bethlem, 1980). They can be seen in both Type 1 and Type 2 fibres and even in the intrafusal muscle fibres of the muscle spindles. In enzyme histochemical preparations, they are non-reactive, appearing as pale areas. In most cases the presence of rod bodies is the only abnormality in the muscle biopsy, but in some cases scattered small fibres may be seen with increased central nucleation. Rod bodies may coexist with cores (Afifi *et al*, 1965) and with failure of fibre type differentiation (Nienhuis *et al.*, 1967).

Ultrastructural studies (Fig. 7.2) show the rods to be rectangular and electron-dense. When situated in the myofibrils of a fibre they usually occupy a single sarcomere and seem to originate from the Z-bands of affected sarcomeres, but when found at the periphery of a fibre they lie in various orientations in granular cytoplasm without attachment to myofilaments. Their protein composition is uncertain but they react in histochemical preparations for tyrosine and are thought to consist of tropomyosin or actinin.

Rod bodies are a non-specific feature of degenerative change in myofibrils, and are seen in a number of different disorders including many other myopathies and neurogenic disorders (Swash and Schwartz, 1981a). In these disorders rod bodies are usually found in myofilaments and not in a subsarcolemmal location. They are also found in normal external ocular muscles.

7.2   Central core disease

Central cores, multicores (minicores) and focal loss of cross-striations are related abnormalities which are difficult to classify separately since they may all occur in the same biopsy (Bethlem *et al.*, 1978; Swash and Schwartz, 1981b). However, these abnormalities are usually regarded as pathognomonic of separate entities because each of these pathological features may occur alone, and because the clinical features, especially the occurrence of associated ophthalmoplegia in cases with focal loss of cross-striations, vary from case to case. Central core disease was the first of the benign myopathies of childhood to be recognized. The major features consist of hypotonia, delay in achieving motor milestones and mild, non-progressive weakness (Shy and Magee, 1956) sometimes

Fig. 7.1 (a) Nemaline myopathy. × 560; Gomori trichrome, longitudinal section. Child aged 2 years. The characteristic rod bodies are located in the subsarcolemmal region. They are arranged in clumps; note their small size, and the absence of other abnormality in the fibres. (b) Transverse section of same case as (a). × 617. (c) Rod bodies. × 350; Gomori trichrome. In this adult muscle the rod bodies were a non-specific and less prominent abnormality than in the typical infantile onset cases.

associated with skeletal abnormalities. Central core disease is usually a dominantly inherited disorder.

7.2.1 Muscle biopsy

In central core disease there is an abnormal central, or somewhat eccentric, zone within the transverse area of affected fibres. This zone shows reduced or absent oxidative enzyme activity, e.g. NADH (Fig. 7.3), and reduced reactivity in PAS preparations. In Gomori preparations this abnormal zone stains bluish but in HE the core region usually appears normal although it can be recognized with phase contrast microscopy. Most cores occur in Type 1 fibres. In ATPase preparations (pH 4.3) the core regions may be reactive or unreactive. This difference has led to subdivision of the core abnormality into structured and unstructured types (Neville, 1978).

In structured cores the core region shows a normal or increased reaction with ATPase; and with the electron microscope this zone shows myofilaments slightly more contracted than in the surrounding normal area of the fibre. The Z-bands are irregular, widened or smeared, and mitochondria are absent.

Fig. 7.2 Rod bodies. EM, × 21 000. The rod bodies are seen as granular electron-dense bodies with sharp borders, arising from Z-band material. In conditions other than nemaline myopathy, rod bodies often occur in association with zones of myofibrillar degeneration.

Fig. 7.3 Cores. × 560; NADH, Longitudinal section. In this biopsy core-like zones of non-reactivity are present. These contain degenerate myofibrils, and mitochondria are absent. In central core disease this abnormality (unstructured cores) extends through long segments of affected fibres, but in this case the abnormality is discrete. The latter is more typical of multicore disease. The slit-like zones of unreactivity are termed 'focal loss of cross-striations'.

In unstructured cores there is loss of the normal myofibrillar pattern, and of mitochondria, so that the regular striated appearance is lost and the ATPase reaction is negative. Unstructured cores resemble the early stage of target fibre formation (Fig. 7.4) and there is confusion in the nomenclature of these abnormalities (Schmitt and Volk, 1975; Swash and Schwartz, 1981a; b).

Cores are usually said to extend through the length of affected fibres without interruption, but most longitudinal sections do not extend more than a few hundred micrometers at the most, and this is therefore a difficult point of which to be certain. By contrast, *multi (mini) cores* occur at multiple zones in the transverse area of affected fibres, usually Type 1 fibres, and extend only a short longitudinal distance. The edges of the lesions are sharply circumscribed. Central nucleation is more frequent in biopsies showing multicores than in central core disease itself. *Focal loss of cross-striations* (van Wijngaarden *et al.*, 1977) is a less common abnormality (Fig. 7.5), consisting of a linear transverse lucency in NADH preparations, resembling unstructured cores, but extending only a few sarcomeres in the length of the fibre (Fig. 7.6) (Swash and Schwartz, 1981b).

Fig. 7.4 Core or target? × 360; NADH. There is a pale, non-reactive zone in the pale Type 2 fibre at the top of the illustration which resembles a core. However, there is also a small cluster of NADH-dark, pointed, atrophic denervated fibres, suggesting denervation and thus implying that the 'core' is really a target (see text). A nearby dark Type 1 fibre shows a small central target-like abnormality.

Fig. 7.5 Focal loss of cross-striations. × 532; Toluidine blue. The focal zone of loss of cross-striations is clearly evident in this semithin plastic-embedded section.

Fig. 7.6 Multicore disease. EM, × 8400. This unstructured core consists of a zone of disrupted myofilamentous and tubular material, lacking mitochondria. There is a relatively sudden transition to normal muscle at the edges of the lesion.

7.3 Myotubular (centronuclear) myopathy

In the severe form of this disorder, cardiopulmonary problems, together with facial and bulbar weakness, often lead to death in the first two years of life, but less severe forms of the disease, even presenting in adult life may occur. External ophthalmoplegia is often a feature of the childhood-onset cases. The pattern of inheritance is variable.

7.3.1 *Muscle biopsy*

The main abnormality is the presence of central nuclei in zones of affected fibres devoid of ATPase reactivity (Fig. 7.7). This central zone contains aggregates of mitochondria but few myofibrils. Type 1 fibres are affected more severely than Type 2 fibres. These fibres resemble fetal myotubes (Spiro *et al.*, 1966) but not all fibres show this perinuclear, clear zone and the term centronuclear myopathy is often preferred to myotubular myopathy.

Fig. 7.7 (a) Myotubular myopathy. × 350; ATPase, pH 4.3. Many of the fibres contain a central zone of non-reactivity, corresponding to the nucleus, and a perinuclear zone of absence of myofibrils. Note the small-sized muscle fibres characteristic of biopsies at this age (1 year). (b) HE and (c) ATPase, pH 9.5, × 427. Normal fetal myotubes. Abortion at 2 months gestation. In the limb the developing muscles are represented by clusters of normal myotubes. Their tubular form is seen in the ATPase preparation (c) and their central nuclei in the longitudinal HE stain (b). This stage of development is followed by maturation so that at birth myotubes are not normally present.

(b)

(c)

7.4 Congenital fibre-type disproportion

This disorder presents with hypotonia, weakness and respiratory difficulties. Contractures and congenital dislocation of the hip are features of the disease (Cavanagh *et al.*, 1979). Inheritance may be dominant or recessive.

7.4.1 Muscle biopsy

In this disorder there is disproportion in the diameters of Type 1 and Type 2 fibres (Brooke, 1973). This disparity is due to hypertrophy of Type 2 fibres, especially Type 2B fibres, the Type 1 fibres being of normal size (Fig. 7.8). In order to establish the diagnosis the mean diameter of Type 1 fibres should be at least 12% less than that of the Type 2 fibres (Swash and Schwartz, 1981a). Associated abnormalities, including increased central nucleation, moth-eaten fibres and rod bodies may also occur.

The disorder must be differentiated from Type 1 atrophy found in myotonic dystrophy and myotubular myopathy. The histological features may also sometimes resemble those found in the early stages of Werdnig–Hoffmann disease (Type 1 spinal muscular atrophy) but in the latter, fibre-type grouping is usually a feature and the large fibres in the latter condition may be undifferentiated.

Fig. 7.8 Fibre-type disproportion. × 350; ATPase, pH 4.3. The pale Type 2 fibres are large and rounded. There is Type 1 fibre predominance but the Type 1 fibres are of a uniformly small size.

Fig. 7.9 Tubular aggregates. EM, × 70 200. Affected fibres show a peripheral, bright red, inclusion in the Gomori preparation consisting of stacked tubules derived from the sarcoplasmic reticulum. This abnormality is a non-specific finding. In this EM preparation the stacked tubular structure of this inclusion can be seen.

130 Biopsy Pathology of Muscle

7.5 Myopathy with tubular aggregates

Tubular aggregates are a rare phenomenon found most abundantly in patients with periodic paralysis but also reported in myotonia congenita. A few cases of mild weakness with hypotonia in infancy have also been reported in which tubular aggregates, usually restricted to Type 2B fibres but occasionally also found in Type 1 fibres (Dobkin and Verity, 1978) were the only abnormality. Tubular aggregates consist of clusters of closely packed tubules (Fig. 7.9), probably derived from the sarcoplasmic reticulum, which stain bright red in Gomori stains and which react positively in NADH preparations but negatively in SDH preparations.

7.6 Failure of fibre-type differentiation

In this rare disorder the muscle fibres fail to differentiate into fibre types in the ATPase preparations. Sometimes myopathic features may be present, for example, fat 'replacement' may be a feature.

7.7 Other benign myopathies of childhood

A number of other, extremely rare disorders without specific clinical features are recognized by their histological or ultrastructural appearances, for example, subsarcolemmal finger-print inclusions (Engel et al., 1972), zebra body myopathy (Lake and Wilson, 1975), etc (see Mastaglia and Hudgson, 1981, for review).

7.8 Congenital muscular dystrophy

This term is used to describe children in whom a non-progressive congenital myopathy with severe weakness, often associated with arthrogryposis, is accompanied by histological appearances in the muscle biopsy typical of muscular dystrophy. There may be severe abnormality in the muscle biopsy, consisting of fibrosis and fat replacement, with marked variability in fibre size, although usually without active fibre necrosis and regeneration. The blood CK level, unlike that found in Duchenne muscular dystrophy is normal or only slightly raised (Donner et al., 1975). In other cases only minimal pathological change may be found (Dubowitz, 1978).

References

Afifi, A. K., Smith, T. W. and Zellweger, H. (1965), Congenital non-progressive myopathy: central core and nemaline myopathy in one family. *Neurology (Minneap.)*, **15**, 371–81.

Bethlem, J. (1980), *Myopathies*, 2nd edn, Elsevier, Amsterdam.
Bethlem, J., Arts, W. F. and Dingemans, K. P. (1978), Common origin of rods, cores, miniature cores and focal loss of cross-striations. *Arch. Neurol.*, **35**, 555–66.
Brooke, M. H. (1973), Congenital fibre type disproportion. In *Clinical Studies in Myology* (ed. B. A. Kakulas), Excerpta Medica, Amsterdam, pp. 147–59.
Cavanagh, N. P. C., Lake, B. D. and McMeniman, P. (1979), Congenital fibre type disproportion myopathy: a histological diagnosis with an uncertain clinical outlook. *Arch. Dis. Child.*, **54**, 735–43.
Dobkin, B. H. and Verity, M. A. (1978), Familial neuromuscular disease with Type 1 fibre hypoplasia, tubular aggregates, cardiomyopathy and myasthenic features. *Neurology (NY)*, **28**, 1135–40.
Donner, M. Rapola, J. and Somer, H. (1975), Congenital muscular dystrophy: a clinico-pathological and follow-up study of 15 patients. *Neuropëdiatrie*, **6**, 239–58.
Dubowitz, V (1978), *Muscle Disorders in Childhood*, W. B. Saunders, London.
Dubowitz, V. (1980), *The Floppy Infant Syndrome*, 2nd edn, Heinemann, London.
Engel, A. G., Angelini, C. and Gomez, M. R. (1972), Finger print body myopathy. *Mayo Clin. Proc.*, **47**, 377–88.
Hudgson, P., Gardner-Medwin, D., Fulthorpe, J. L. and Walton, J. N. (1967), Nemaline myopathy. *Neurology (Minneap.)*, **17**, 1125–42.
Lake, B. D. and Wilson, T. (1975), Zebra body myopathy: clinical, histochemical and ultrastructural studies. *J. Neurol. Sci.*, **24**, 437–46.
Lundberg, A. (1979), Dissociated motor development; developmental patterns, clinical characteristics; causal factors and outcome with special reference to late-walking children. *Neuropëdiatrie*, **10**, 161–82.
Mastaglia, F. L. and Hudgson, P. (1981), Ultrastructural studies of diseased muscle. In *Disorders of Voluntary Muscle*, 4th edn (ed. J. N. Walton), Churchill Livingstone, Edinburgh, pp. 296–356.
Neville, H. E. (1978); Ultrastructural changes in diseases of human skeletal muscle. In *Handbook of Clinical Neurology*, Vol. 40 (eds P. J. Vinken and G. W. Bruyn), North Holland, Amsterdam, pp. 63–124.
Nienhuis, A. W., Coleman, F. R., Brown, W. J. et al. (1967), Nemaline myopathy: a histopathologic and biochemical study. *Am. J. Clin. Pathol.*, **48**, 1–13.
Paine, R. S. (1963), The future of the floppy infant, a follow up study of 133 patients *Dev. Med. Child. Neurol.*, **5**, 115–24.
Schmitt, H. P. and Volk, B. (1975), The relationship between target, targetoid and targetoid-core fibres in severe neurogenic muscular atrophy. *J. Neurol.*, **210**, 167–81.
Shy, G. M. and Magee, K. R. (1956), A new congenital non progressive myopathy. *Brain*, **79**, 610–21.
Spiro, A. J., Shy, G. M. and Gonatas, N. K. (1966), Myotubular myopathy. *Arch. Neurol.*, **14**, 1–14.
Swash, M. and Schwartz, M. S. (1981a), *Neuromuscular Diseases: A Practical Approach to Diagnosis and Management*, Springer-Verlag, Berlin, Heidelberg, New York.
Swash, M. and Schwartz, M. S. (1981b), Familial multicore disease with focal loss of cross striations and ophthalmoplegia. *J. Neurol. Sci.*, **52**, 1–10.
van Wijngaarden, G. K., Bethlem, J., Dingemans, K. P. et al. (1977), Familial focal loss of cross-striations. *J. Neurol.*, **216**, 163–72.

8 Metabolic, endocrine and drug-induced myopathies

The metabolic, endocrine and drug-induced myopathies are discussed in this chapter as a related group of disorders because, in a general sense, they share a common pathogenetic mechanism. The metabolic myopathies result from a biochemical defect in muscle metabolism itself, the endocrine myopathies from an abnormal hormonal environment, probably affecting muscle metabolism, and the drug-induced myopathies from a direct toxic effect of the drug on muscle metabolism. In some drug-induced myopathies, e.g. malignant hyperpyrexia myopathy, the drug effect is manifest only in susceptible individuals.

8.1 Metabolic myopathies

The clinical features of this group of disorders vary considerably. Their severity ranges from benign muscle cramps to a presentation resembling the limb-girdle syndrome with marked muscular atrophy. In some instances acute episodes of myoglobinuria may occur, and in others, e.g. the periodic paralyses, attacks of severe flaccid weakness with rapid recovery are a feature. Exercise may precipitate symptoms in many of these metabolic disorders. The main types of metabolic myopathy are shown in Table 8.1.

It should be noted that several of the major types of metabolic myopathy are characterized histologically by major abnormalities in muscle fibres. For example, in those glycogenoses in which a myopathy is a feature glycogen is stored in muscle fibres; in the mitochondrial myopathies the mitochondria show characteristic abnormalities in number, distribution and ultrastructure (ragged-red fibres); in the lipid storage myopathies neutral lipid accumulates in muscle fibres; in the periodic paralyses, muscle fibres are often vacuolated in biopsies taken during a period of weakness.

Table 8.1 Metabolic myopathies

Glycogenoses affecting muscle
  Type II : acid maltase deficiency
  Type III: debranching enzyme deficiency
  Type IV: branching enzyme deficiency
  Type V : myophosphorylase deficiency
  Type VII: phosphofructokinase deficiency

Mitochondrial myopathies
  Disorders of the electron transport chain

Lipid storage myopathies
  Carnitine deficiency
  Systemic and muscle forms
  (Carnitine palmityl transferase deficiency)

Periodic paralysis
  Hypokalaemic
  Hyperkalaemic
  Normokalaemic
  Thyrotoxic
  Secondary hypokalaemic and hyperkalaemic muscular weakness

Malignant hyperpyrexia myopathy

Myoglobinurias

8.1.1   Glycogenoses

Only five of the known forms of glycogenosis are associated with muscular involvement. In Type I glycogenosis (glucose 6 phosphatase deficiency) hypotonia occurs; this is probably secondary to lactic acidosis since glucose 6 phosphatase is not normally present in skeletal muscle. All the glycogenoses are inherited as autosomal recessive disorders, but genetic heterogeneity is a feature of all of them.

(a) *Type II glycogenosis (acid maltase deficiency)*. Two forms of this disease occur. In the infantile form (Pompe's disease) there is generalized muscular weakness, with hypotonia, cardiomegaly and hepatomegaly, respiratory difficulties and enlargement of the tongue (Hogan, *et al.*, 1969). The adult form resembles the limb–girdle dystrophy syndrome, presenting in adult life as a slowly progressive myopathy sometimes with calf hypertrophy (Engel, 1970a). An intermediate form, beginning in childhood, has also been described. The infantile and adult forms may occur in the same family (Busch *et al*, 1979).

Muscle biopsy. The muscle fibres are rounded and show increased variability in size. There may be increased endomysial fibrous tissue. The major feature is the presence of PAS-positive vacuoles within muscle fibres. These vacuoles are usually multiple and very small. Their PAS-positive material is diastase-digestible and they are strongly reactive for acid phosphatase indicating that they are autophagic vacuoles derived from lysosomes (Engel, 1970a). In the adult form (Fig. 8.1) small angular fibres and fibre-type grouping, thought to indicate

(a)

(b)

Fig. 8.1 Glycogen storage myopathy. (Type II glycogenosis; adult-onset type.) (a) × 350; HE. Two fibres show prominent vacuolization, and two contain central nuclei. (b) × 350; PAS. The vacuoles in the fibres (in another part of the biopsy) are PAS positive. (c) × 350; acid phosphatase. The vacuoles are filled with punctate positive reactivity indicative of lysosomal activity. (d) × 140; ATPase, pH 4.3. The vacuoles mainly affect fibres of intermediate type, but Type 2A fibres are also affected.

anterior horn cell involvement, have been reported (Karpati *et al.*, 1977). The biopsy is most abnormal in more severely affected muscles, and increased acid phosphatase activity may be found in fibres apparently devoid of vacuoles. In infantile cases all muscle fibres contain vacuoles.

In ultrastructural studies most of the vacuoles are membrane-bound or consist of autophagic vacuoles. Glycogen is found in both these sites, but is also present in increased quantity free in the sarcoplasm, between the myofibrils.

(b) *Type III glycogenosis (debranching enzyme deficiency)*. In one form of the disease hepatomegaly, retardation of growth and attacks of hypoglycaemia are common, but myopathy is slight, and in the other there is a prominent myopathy beginning in childhood or adult life, with progressive muscular weakness and hepatomegaly. Excessive fatiguability may be prominent (Brunberg *et al.*, 1971). There is electrocardiographic evidence of cardiac involvement.

Muscle biopsy. There is a marked vacuolar myopathy. The vacuoles contain glycogen but are negative for acid phosphatase and the glycogen granules are not membrane bound. Sarcoplasmic glycogen is also increased. No neurogenic component has been reported (Di Mauro *et al.*, 1979).

(c) *Type IV glycogenosis (branching enzyme deficiency)*. Muscle weakness and atrophy is a mild feature of some patients with this disorder. Hepatosplenomegaly and failure to thrive are the main features. The disorder is extremely rare, affecting infants. An adult form probably also occurs (Tarvik *et al.*, 1974). The biopsy shows a vacuolar myopathy in which only scattered fibres are affected.

(d) *Type V glycogenosis (myophosphorylase deficiency)*. This is the commonest and the best known of the muscle glycogenoses (McArdle, 1951). The disorder may begin at any age but it is commonest in young adults. It presents with weakness, fatiguability and muscular cramps after exercise. Myoglobinuria may be a feature. At rest there is usually no clinical abnormality, although in longstanding cases muscular weakness and wasting may develop. Following ischaemic exercise there is little or no rise in the venous blood lactate or pyruvate levels. This abnormality is not specific for McArdle's disease since it is also found in phosphofructo-kinase deficiency. A severe infantile form has been reported.

Muscle biopsy. Myophosphorylase is absent from the biopsy (Fig. 8.2), except in regenerating fibres in which the fetal form of the enzyme can be detected (Di Mauro *et al.*, 1978). The muscle biopsy shows little other abnormality, apart from subsarcolemmal accumulations of PAS-positive glycogen, appearing as pink blebs (Fig. 8.3). Necrotic fibres, small atrophic fibres and scattered regenerating fibres may be prominent in biopsies taken soon after severe exertion and in longstanding cases. There may be increased central nucleation (Dubowitz and Brooke, 1973). Ultrastructural studies show increased

Fig. 8.2   McArdle's disease (Type V glycogenosis). (a) × 350. Myophosphorylase activity in normal muscle. (b) × 140. Absence of detectable myophosphorylase reactivity in McArdle's disease.

Fig. 8.3 McArdle's disease. × 350; PAS. There is unusually prominent glycogen, particularly in Type 1 fibres.

glycogen content in the intermyofibrillar sarcoplasm. It has been noted in some cases that individual muscles may show decreased, and others absent phosphorylase activity. Smooth muscle is not involved, and the heart is also spared.

(e) *Type VII glycogenosis (phosphofructokinase deficiency)*. This rare disorder clinically resembles McArdle's disease, although muscular weakness is somewhat more prominent. The ischaemic exercise test is useful since, as in McArdle's disease, there is no rise in venous lactate or pyruvate after the period of ischaemic work. Red cell phosphofructokinase levels may be decreased and haemolytic disease has been noted (Tarui *et al.*, 1969).

Muscle biopsy. There is variation in fibre diameter, subsarcolemmal accumulation of glycogen, and a few necrotic fibres may be found (Tobin *et al.*, 1973). The absence of muscle phosphofructokinase can be demonstrated by an enzyme histochemical reaction (Bonilla and Schotland, 1970).

8.1.2 *Mitochondrial myopathies*

The term mitochondrial myopathy is used to describe a group of disorders characterized by abnormalities in the morphology of mitochondria in muscle fibres. In many cases the mitochondrial abnormality has been correlated with biochemical abnormalities in mitochondrial enzyme reactions. Most of these cases have been sporadic or have shown autosomal recessive inheritance. Similar morphological changes in mitochondria occur in patients with oculo-cranio-somatic syndrome, a complex, familial, system degeneration of the nervous system, in which muscle involvement may occur. In most of the latter the underlying biochemical abnormality remains unknown.

(a) *Clinical features.* Several clinical syndromes are recognized. In many patients, especially those presenting before the age of 20, there is a progressive ophthalmoplegia, often associated with mild proximal muscle weakness, and sometimes also with other features, e.g. cerebellar ataxia, cardiomyopathy with conduction block, retinal degeneration, mental retardation, sensory deafness and short stature (Kearns–Sayre syndrome; see Berenberg et al., 1977). In others the clinical presentation is with slowly progressive proximal weakness, often without marked wasting, but usually with prominent fatiguability and reduced exercise tolerance. Muscle cramps, or even myoglobinuria, may be a feature.

(b) *Pathological features.* Despite the various clinical presentations and the differing biochemical abnormalities most of these disorders show similar morphological changes in the muscle biopsy. The abnormality can almost invariably be recognized by light microscopy, without recourse to the electron microscope. The term ragged-red fibre is often used to describe the characteristic abnormality (Engel, 1971). Ragged-red fibres (Fig. 8.4) consist of fibres in which there is an irregular subsarcolemmal rim of bright red or reddish blue material in the Gomori trichrome stain. The abnormality is often patchily distributed through the cross-sectional area of the affected fibre. The abnormal material is positive in the oxidative enzyme reactions, e.g. NADH or SDH, faintly basophilic, usually positive for neutral lipid, and unreactive for ATPase. The most specific of these reactions is the SDH technique, since a positive reaction for this enzyme reaction is firm evidence for the presence of accumulations of mitochondria (Fig. 8.5). The ragged-red fibre abnormality particularly affects Type 1 muscle fibres (Olson, et al., 1972), and these abnormal Type I fibres are almost always smaller than the unaffected Type I fibres (Swash et al., 1978). Generally, there is little other abnormality, although there may be some increase in central nucleation, and some small angulated fibres and fibres showing a moth-eaten appearance in NADH reactions may be seen. Necrotic and regenerating fibres, and interstitial fibrosis are not features of most of these disorders. However, a marked increase in the size and number of neutral lipid droplets, together with increased glycogen content, may be a prominent feature, especially in patients with muscle carnitine deficiency (Engel and Angelini, 1973). Lipid accumulates mainly in Type I fibres.

Although ragged-red fibres have come to be regarded as a specific feature of mitochondrial myopathies, in which they are prominent, occurring in as many as 20% of Type I fibres, single, isolated ragged-red fibres may sometimes be found in a variety of other disorders, e.g. polymyositis and limb–girdle dystrophy, in which a primary mitochondrial disorder is not suspected. In order to suggest a diagnosis of

(a)

(b)

Fig. 8.4 Ragged-red fibres in a mitochondrial myopathy. × 600. (a) Gomori trichrome. The characteristic change is a peripheral, red-staining, zone, with a granular appearance to the fibre itself. (b) NADH. The peripheral zone is faintly positive with zones of non-reactivity. (c) ATPase, pH 4.3. The peripheral zone is non-reactive.

Fig. 8.5 Ragged-red fibres in cytochrome b deficiency. × 427; SDH. The mitochondrial-rich peripheral zone reacts darkly; the abnormal fibres are virtually all Type 1 fibres.

mitochondrial myopathy ragged-red fibres should be the main pathological feature (Fig. 8.5), and other structural changes should be relatively
minor (Olson *et al.*, 1972).

With the electron microscope the mitochondrial abnormality can be
further characterized (Tassin *et al.*, 1980). Subsarcolemmal and intermyofibrillar aggregates of mitochondria are seen (Fig. 8.6). These
mitochondria are usually larger than normal, and abnormalities in their

Fig. 8.6 Mitochondrial myopathy. Ragged-red fibres. EM, × 26125. The
mitochondria contain eosinophilic dense bodies, or paracrystalline material and
their cristae are absent.

cristae are prominent. Paracrystalline inclusions are particularly characteristic (Fig. 8.7), consisting of rectangular or curvilinear arrays of
membranes arranged in a linear or grid-like pattern of about 20 nm

Fig. 8.7   EM, × 23 100. Paracrystalline inclusions in mitochondria in a ragged-red
fibre.

separation. These inclusions are frequently multiple and arranged in parallel rows – the 'parking-lot' inclusions. They can usually be seen to be situated between the displaced inner and outer membranes of the mitochondrion, and are often attached to these membranes by short transverse bridges of membranous material. Mitochondria containing paracrystalline inclusions are usually devoid of cristae. Other mitochondria show degraded cristae, or whorls of parallel membranes. Osmiophilic dense bodies, and glycogen granules, are also often found within the abnormal mitochondria in these disorders (Tassin and Brucher, 1982).

The myofibrillar architecture also shows abnormalities, with disarray or even fragmentation of myofibrils. There are increased amounts of sarcoplasmic glycogen, and lipid droplets are also unusually prominent.

(c) *Biochemical characterization*. The mitochondrial myopathies reflect the morphological expression of biochemical defects in metabolic pathways involving oxidative, mitochondrial-dependent processes. A number of genetically discrete abnormalities in the electron transport, flavoprotein chain have recently been characterized and in each of these disorders the morphological abnormality, both by light and electron microscope, has been similar to that described above. Mitochondrial abnormalities of this type also occur in disorders of transport of metabolites into mitochondria, e.g. carnitine deficiency; in this instance muscle lipid droplet deposition is particularly prominent. These disorders have recently been reviewed by Morgan-Hughes (1982) and Morgan-Hughes *et al.*, (1982).

8.1.3   *Lipid storage myopathies*

This term has been used to describe accumulation of neutral lipid in muscle fibres. It is thus a non-specific abnormality. Harriman and Reid (1972) reviewed 139 cases in which excess lipid droplets were noted. These droplets were located principally in Type 1 fibres. The most common disorders showing this abnormality were steroid myopathy and alcoholic myopathy. Diabetic neuropathy and myasthenia gravis were also sometimes associated with increased lipid droplet formation. Excess lipid droplets in Type 2 fibres are rare.

Lipid droplets are a prominent feature in Type 1 and Type 2A fibres in *carnitine deficiency*. This disorder occurs in several forms. In the adult onset variety the disorder is limited to skeletal muscle, and lipid droplet accumulation (Fig. 8.8), with ragged-red fibres and mitochondrial abnormalities, are diagnostic features of the muscle biopsy (Willner *et al.*, 1979). In childhood a severe systemic form of carnitine deficiency in which myopathy is associated with hepatomegaly, metabolic acidosis, encephalopathy and cardiomyopathy has been reported; the muscle biopsy shows similar features to the adult onset disorder (Karpati *et al.*, 1975). In carnitine palmityl transferase deficiency, a disorder presenting with cramps, muscular pain and myoglobinuria, the muscle biopsy shows little abnormality apart from a slight excess of lipid droplets (Bank *et al.*, 1975). Muscle carnitine deficiency may also develop in starvation and in chronic haemodialysis, but little is known of the histological features in the muscle biopsy in these patients. Lipid droplets are also prominent in the mitochondrial myopathies themselves (see above).

8.1.4 *Periodic paralysis*

This term refers to a group of disorders characterized by episodic and often asymmetrical limb–girdle weakness, with recovery between attacks. Attacks may last for several hours. There is usually an autosomal dominant pattern of inheritance. The commonest form is associated with *hypokalaemia* during attacks of weakness, but *hyperkalaemic* and *normokalaemic* forms have been described (see Swash and Schwartz, 1981, for review).

In all three varieties of familial periodic paralysis the muscle biopsy shows only slight abnormalities between attacks but in biopsies taken during an episode of weakness vacuolar change is prominent (Fig. 8.9). These vacuoles vary in size but do not deform the external shape of the fibre. They appear empty or faintly PAS positive. In patients who have sustained severe or prolonged weakness calcium salts may be deposited in the region of these vacuoles (Weller and McArdle, 1971). The vacuoles are unreactive for acid phosphatase, but affected fibres sometimes show faint or patchy basophilia. During the recovery phase the biopsy may contain a few necrotic fibres undergoing phagocytosis, and regenerating fibres may also be recognized.

In patients in whom multiple attacks of weakness have occurred during many years, mild proximal weakness may be persistent and this is usually associated with histological features of a myopathy, including increased variability in fibre size, increased central nucleation and isolated necrotic and regenerating fibres, but even in these cases the presence of scattered vacuolated fibres should suggest the diagnosis.

Electron microscopy (Fig. 8.10) of vacuolated fibres reveals that the vacuoles, which are lined by a single layer of membrane, are continuous with dilated tubules of the sarcoplasmic reticulum (Engel, 1970b). The vacuoles often contain amorphous material, thought to consist of mucopolysaccharide. The sarcoplasm is normal but focal areas of myofibrillar disruption and repair are common. Similar vacuoles occur in other hypokalaemic myopathies, e.g. those associated with alcoholism (Rubenstein and Wainapel, 1977), liquorice toxicity and diuretic abuse.

8.15   *Malignant hyperpyrexia myopathy*

Although this disorder represents a metabolic myopathy the clinical features become apparent only after exposure to certain drugs, e.g. anaesthetic drugs. The trait is inherited in an autosomal dominant pattern. Susceptible individuals can sometimes be detected by the presence of a raised blood CK, but an *in vitro* test of muscle metabolism in

(c)

Fig. 8.8 Muscle carnitine deficiency of adult-onset. (a) × 350; HE. The striking abnormality is the presence of unstained, rounded lipid vacuoles of varying size, more prominent in some fibres than in others. These differ from ice-crystals in their distribution, size and shape. (b) × 350; Oil red O. The vacuoles seen in the HE stain are stained intensely in this neutral lipid preparation. (c) × 350; ATPase, pH 4.3. The lipid droplets are unreactive, and are found mainly in Type 1 fibres.

Fig. 8.9 Hypokalaemic periodic paralysis. × 350; HE. There is slight variability in fibre size with increased central nucleation. One fibre shows a prominent vacuolar zone, accompanied by central nucleation.

Fig. 8.10   EM. Hypokalaemic periodic paralysis. The origin of the vacuoles, lined by a single-layered membrane, from the tubular system can be seen. There is some disorganization of the myofibrillar pattern in this region.

the presence of low concentrations of anaesthetic agents, especially halothane, in which muscle contraction occurs in abnormal individuals, is far more reliable (Ellis and Halsall, 1980).

The muscle biopsy is usually abnormal; there are features of a mild non-progressive myopathy consisting of increased variability in fibre size, increased central nucleation, rare split fibres and some moth-eaten fibres. In some cases the histological features of central core disease have been reported (Denborough *et al.*, 1973). In acute episodes muscle fibre necrosis may be found, but there is often little abnormality apart from reduced glycogen content, a dilated tubular system and ruptured mitochondria (Schiller and Mair, 1974).

8.1.6   Myoglobinurias

Generally, myoglobinuria is a feature associated with acute, massive muscle cell necrosis. It is therefore found in a wide variety of muscular disorders (Table 8.2). Myoglobin is a protein with a relatively low

Table 8.2 Causes of myoglobinuria

Idiopathic paroxysmal myoglobinuria

Metabolic
  (a) Myophosphorylase deficiency (Glycogenosis Type V: McArdle's syndrome)
  (b) Phosphofructokinase deficiency (Glycogenosis Type VII)
  (c) Hypokalaemic periodic paralysis
  (d) Carnitine palmityl transferase deficiency
  (e) Malignant hyperpyrexia myopathy
  (f) Other systemic disorders, e.g. diabetic acidosis

Toxic
  (a) Alcohol, carbon monoxide and barbiturate poisoning
  (b) Liquorice excess (hypokalaemia)
  (c) Heroin myopathy
  (d) Chloroquine, amphotericin B and epsilon amino caproic acid-induced acute
      toxic myopathies
  (e) Exposure to industrial toxins (Haff's disease)
  (f) Various biological toxins, e.g. hornet stings, Malaysian sea-snake bites, etc.
  (g) Heat stroke and high fever

Trauma and ischaemia
  (a) Crush injuries
  (b) Volkmann's ischaemic contracture
  (c) Anterior tibial syndrome ('shin splints')
  (d) Major arterial occlusion
  (e) Severe, prolonged exercise

Acute polymyositis and acute necrotizing myopathy associated with carcinoma

Postinfectious(viruses)
  (a) Influenza A
  (b) Coxsackie
  (c) *Herpes simplex*
  (d) Epstein Barr

---

molecular weight (17,000 Dalton), and a low renal threshold. Urinary myoglobin reacts positively with benzidine, but can often be detected clinically by the characteristic brown colour. A sensitive immunoprecipitation method has recently supplanted the benzidine method (Markowitz and Wobig, 1977). Attacks of myoglobinuria are often associated clinically with muscle weakness, pain and muscle swelling. In idiopathic myoglobinuria the attacks follow strenuous exercise, usually in young men (Type 1), or may be related to other unknown factors (Type 2).

The muscle biopsy in any myoglobinuric syndrome may show widespread acute muscle fibre necrosis. Regenerating fibres are often prominent, usually consisting of subsarcolemmal crescents of basophilic sarcoplasm of varying size, containing multiple lipid droplets. There may be a sparse lymphocytic infiltrate. The basic fascicular structure of the muscle is maintained, and histological recovery is usually complete unless recurrent attacks occur.

8.2 Endocrine myopathies

Myopathies are common features of endocrine disease (Table 8.3) but muscular involvement is comparatively rarely of clinical significance. Muscular symptoms may, however, be a presenting feature in hyperthyroidism or in myxoedema, and sometimes also in disorders of calcium metabolism. Steroid myopathy is a common iatrogenic disorder, and a relatively late complication of Cushing's disease.

Table 8.3 Endocrine myopathies

Thyroid myopathies
  Thyrotoxicosis
  Myxoedema

Parathyroid disorders and osteomalacia
  Hypoparathyroidism
  Hyperparathyroidism
  Osteomalacia

Andrenal disorders (and steroid myopathy)
  Addison's disease
  Cushing's syndrome
  Steroid therapy

Pituitary disorders
  Acromegaly

The CK may be greatly raised in some patients with myxoedema (McKeran et al., 1980) although moderately increased levels are more common. In the other endocrine myopathies the CK is usually normal, although it may be slightly raised in some patients with acromegaly.

8.2.1 Muscle pathology

The histological changes in the muscle in endocrine myopathies are generally only slight, even when weakness is quite marked. In acromegaly Type 1 fibres are usually slightly hypertrophied and Type 2 fibres, especially Type 2A fibres, slightly atrophic (Nagulesparen et al., 1976) but some hypertrophied Type 2 fibres may also be present. Necrotic muscle

Fig. 8.11 Steroid myopathy. × 350; HE. There is atrophy of some fibres.

Fig. 8.12 Steroid myopathy. × 350; ATPase, pH 9.4. The atrophic fibres are all Type 2 fibres. The paler Type 1 fibres are much less affected.

Fig. 8.13 Alcoholic myopathy. × 140; ATPase, pH 9.4. Prominent Type 2 fibre atrophy.

(a)

(b)

(c)

Fig. 8.14 Epsilon caproic acid myopathy; an acute necrotizing 'toxic' myopathy. (a) × 450; HE. The field consists of necrotic muscle fibres, with peripheral crescents of regeneration. There is a sparse inflammatory cell exudate. (b) × 450; NADH. The regenerating segments are clearly seen in this part of the biopsy. (c) × 450; ATPase, pH 4.3. The regenerating segments show ATPase reactivity, but the necrotic portions of these fibres are unreactive.

fibres are rarely seen (Mastaglia et al., 1970). The muscle fibre hypertrophy may persist even after effective treatment of the acromegaly. In *hypo-* and *hyperparathyroidism* only minimal changes are found in the muscle; Type 2B atrophy has been noted in several studies (Schott and Wills, 1975). The morphological changes in osteomalacia are similarly slight.

In *hyperthyroidism* the main abnormality is atrophy of muscle fibres, but this may be very slight. Focal lymphocytic infiltrates may be present. Muscle fibre necrosis is not a feature, but central nucleation may be excessive. In *myxoedema* light microscopy may reveal some fibre atrophy, increased central nucleation and occasional fibres with subsarcolemmal accumulation of glycogen (McKeran *et al.*, 1980). Degenerating and regenerating fibres are rare (Shirabe *et al.*, 1975). Ultrastructural studies have revealed accumulation of abnormal mitochondria, some containing rectilinear paracrystalline bodies similar to those found in primary mitochondrial myopathies (Godet-Guillain and Fardeau, 1970).

Steroid myopathy shows more marked abnormalities in the muscle biopsy. The main feature is atrophy of both fibre types, particularly of Type 2 fibres (Pleasure *et al.*, 1970). Lipid droplets and glycogen accumulations are prominent, especially in Type 1 fibres. Electron microscopy shows enlarged and degenerate mitochondria, dilatation of the sarcoplasmic reticulum, loss of myofibrils and marked thickening of the basement membrane (Engel, 1966). In the light microscope the Type 2 fibre atrophy may be so prominent that the presence of scattered atrophic fibres in the HE preparation may be interpreted as denervation (Fig. 8.11); however, the limitation of this atrophy to Type 2 fibres in the enzyme histochemical preparation rules out this possibility (Fig. 8.12).

Muscle biopsies are sometimes used to try to assess the possible development of steroid myopathy in patients with polymyositis who have been treated with high-dose steroids for some weeks, yet have remained weak, or even become weaker during treatment. The presence of lipid-laden fibres, especially Type 1 fibres, and of Type 2 fibre atrophy, strongly suggest that steroid myopathy has developed (Askari *et al.*, 1976). The dose of steroid necessary to induce steroid myopathy is variable, e.g. 1.5–6.0 mg dexamethasone daily for 3–12 weeks, and prednisone 15–100 mg daily for periods ranging from 1 month to 5 years (Afifi *et al.*, 1968; Askari *et al.*, 1976).

8.3 Drug-induced myopathies

A large number of different drugs may cause muscular weakness (Swash and Schwartz, 1983). *Painful* proximal myopathies, sometimes associated with myoglobinuria, or with a raised blood CK level, may occur acutely or subacutely. Examples include myopathies associated with alcoholism (Fig. 8.13), emetine and epsilon amino caproic acid treatment. A chronic *painless* myopathy has been described after treatment with chloroquine, perhexilene and steroids, and a similar syndrome may occur in opiate addiction. Repeated intramuscular injection may cause a *focal* myopathy, usually associated with intense local fibrosis. Penicillamine may induce myasthenia gravis or inflammatory myopathy. Hypokalaemia and vacuolar myopathy may follow treatment with diuretics or purgatives. (see p. 145).

In the acute and subacute myopathies fibre necrosis and regeneration may be prominent (Fig. 8.14), and myopathic features may be present in the more chronic drug-induced myopathies. Both perhexilene and chloroquine may cause a vacuolar myopathy. The drug-induced neuromuscular syndromes have been reviewed by Mastaglia and Argov (1981).

References

Afifi, A. K., Bergman, R. A. and Harvey, J. C. (1968), Steroid myopathy: clinical, histological and cytological observations. *Johns Hopkins Med. J.*, **123**, 158–74.

Askari, A., Vignos, P. J. Jr, and Moskowitz, R. W. (1976), Steroid myopathy in connective tissue diseases. *Am. J. Med.*, **61**, 485–92.

Bank, W. J., Di Mauro, S., Bonilla, E. *et al.* (1975), A disorder of lipid metabolism and myoglobinuria. *New Engl. J. Med.*, **292**, 443–9.

Berenberg, R. A., Pellock, J. M., Di Mauro, S. *et al.* (1977), Lumping or splitting? 'Ophthalmoplegia plus' or Kearns-Sayre syndrome? *Ann. Neurol.*, **1**, 37–54.

Bonilla, E. and Schotland, D. L. (1970), Histochemical diagnosis of muscle phosphofructokinase deficiency. *Arch. Neurol.*, **22**, 8–12.

Brunberg, J. A., McCormick, W. F. and Schochet, S. S. (1971), Type III glycogenosis. An adult with diffuse weakness and muscle wasting. *Arch. Neurol.*, **25**, 171–8.

Busch, H. F. M., Koster, J. F. and van Weerden, T. W. (1979), Infantile and adult-onset acid maltase deficiency occurring in the same family. *Neurology (NY)*, **29**, 415–16.

Denborough, M. A., Dennett, X. and Anderson, P. M. (1973), Central core disease and malignant hyperpyrexia. *Br. Med. J.*, **1**, 272–3.

Di Mauro, S., Arnold, S., Miranda, A. and Rowland, L. P. (1978), McArdle's disease: the mystery of reappearing phosphorylase activity in muscle culture – a fetal isoenzyme. *Ann. Neurol.*, **3**, 60–6.

Di Mauro, S., Hartwig, G. B., Hayes, A. *et al.* (1979), Debranching deficiency: neuromuscular disorders in 5 adults. *Ann. Neurol.*, **5**, 422–36.

Dubowitz, V. and Brooke, M. H. (1973), *Muscle Biopsy – A Modern Approach*, W. B. Saunders, London.

Ellis, F. R. and Halsall, P. J. (1980), Malignant hyperpyrexia. *Br. J. Hosp. Med.*, **24**, 318–27.

Engel, A. G. (1966), Electron microscopic observations in thyrotoxic and corticosteroid-induced myopathies. *Mayo Clin. Proc.*, **41**, 785–96.

Engel, A. G. (1970a), Acid maltase deficiency in adults. *Brain*, **93**, 599–606.
Engel, A. G. (1970b), Evolution and content of vacuoles in primary hypokalaemic periodic paralysis. *Mayo Clin. Proc.*, **45**, 774–814.
Engel, A. G. and Angelini, C. (1973), Carnitine deficiency of human muscle with associated lipid storage myopathy: a new syndrome. *Science*, **179**, 899–902.
Engel, W. K. (1971), 'Ragged-red fibres' in ophthalmoplegia syndromes and their differential diagnosis. In *Muscle Diseases* (ed. B. A. Kakulas), ICS 237, Exerpta Medica, Amsterdam, p. 28.
Godet-Guillain, J. and Fardeau, M. (1970), Hypothyroid myopathy: histological and ultrastructural study of an atrophic form. In *Muscle Diseases* (eds J. N. Walton, N. Canal and S. Scarlato), ICS 199, Excerpta Medica, Amsterdam, pp. 512–15.
Harriman, D. G. F. and Reid, R. (1972), The incidence of lipid droplets in human skeletal muscle in neuromuscular disorders: a histochemical, electron microscopic and freeze-etch study. *J. Pathol.*, **106**, 1–24.
Hogan, G. R. Gutamann L., Schmidt, R., and Gilbert, E. (1969), Pompe's disease. *Neurology (Minneap.)*, **19**, 894–900.
Karpati, G., Carpenter, S., Engel, A. G. *et al.* (1975): The syndrome of systemic carnitine deficiency. *Neurology (Minneap.)*, **25**, 16–24.
Karpati, G., Carpenter, S., Eisen, A. *et al.* (1977), The adult form of acid maltase (α 1:4 glucosidase) deficiency. *Ann. Neurol.*, **1**, 276–80.
Markowitz, H. and Wobig, G. H. (1977), Quantitative method for estimating myoglobin in urine. *Clin. Chem.*, **23**, 1689–93.
Mastaglia, F. L. and Argov, Z. (1981), Drug-induced neuromuscular disorders in man. In *Disorders of Voluntary Muscle*, 4th edn (ed. J. N. Walton), Churchill Livingstone, Edinburgh, pp. 873–906.
Mastaglia, F. L., Barwick, D. D. and Hall, R. (1970), Myopathy in acromegaly. *Lancet*, **ii**, 907–9.
McArdle, B. (1951), Myopathy due to a defect in muscle glycogen breakdown. *Clin. Sci.*, **10**, 13–33.
McKeran, R. O., Slavin, G., Ward, P. *et al.* (1980), Hypothyroid myopathy: a clinical and pathological study. *J. Pathol.*, **132**, 35–54.
Morgan-Hughes, J. A. (1982), Defects of the energy pathways of skeletal muscle. In *Recent Advances in Clinical Neurology*, Vol. 3 (eds W. B. Matthews and G. H. Glaser), Churchill Livingstone, Edinburgh., pp. 1–46.
Morgan-Hughes, J. A., Hayes, D. J., Clark, J. B. *et al.* (1982), Mitochondrial encephalomyopathies: biochemical studies in two cases revealed defects in the respiratory chain. *Brain*, **105**, 553–82.
Nagulesparen, M., Trickey, R., Davies, M. J. and Jenkins, J. S. (1976), Muscle changes in acromegaly. *Br. Med. J.*, **2**, 914–15.
Olson, W., Engel, W. K., Walsh, G. O. and Einaugler, R. (1972), Oculo cranio somatic neuromuscular disease with 'ragged-red fibres'. Histochemical and ultrastructural changes in limb muscles of a group of patients with idiopathic progressive external ophthalmoplegia. *Arch. Neurol.*, **26**, 193–211.
Pleasure, D. E., Walsh, G. O. and Engel, W. K. (1970), Atrophy of skeletal muscles in patients with Cushing's syndrome. *Arch. Neurol.*, **22**, 118–25.
Rubenstein, A. E. and Wainapel, S. F. (1977), Acute hypokalaemic myopathy in alcoholism. *Arch. Neurol.*, **34**, 553–5.
Schiller, H. H. and Mair, W. G. P. (1974), Ultrastructural changes of muscle in malignant hyperthermia. *J. Neurol. Sci.*, **21**, 93–100.
Schott, G. D. and Wills, M. R. (1975), Myopathy in hypophosphataemic

osteomalacia presenting in adult life. *J. Neurol. Neurosurg. Psychiatry*, **38**, 297–304.

Shirabe, T., Tawara, S., Terao, A. and Araki, S. (1975), Myxoedematous polyneuropathy. *J. Neurol. Neurosurg. Psychiatry*, **38**, 241–7.

Swash, M. and Schwartz, M. S. (1981), *Neuromuscular Diseases: A Practical Approach to Diagnosis and Management*, Springer-Verlag, Berlin, Heidelberg, New York.

Swash, M. and Schwartz, M. S. (1983) Iatrogenic neuromuscular disorders: a review. *Proc. R. Soc. Med.*, **76**, 149–51.

Swash, M., Schwartz, M. S. and Sargeant, M. K. (1978), The significance of ragged-red fibres in neuromuscular disease. *J. Neurol. Sci.*, **36**, 347–55.

Tarui, S., Kono, N., Nasu, T. and Nishikawa, M. (1969), Enzymatic basis for the co-existence of myopathy and haemolytic disease in inherited muscle phosphofructokinase deficiency. *Biochem. Biophys. Res. Comm.*, **34**, 77–83.

Tarvik, A., Dietrichson, P. K., Svaar, H. and Hudgson, P. (1974), Myopathy with tremor and dementia: a metabolic disorder? *J. Neurol. Sci.*, **21**, 181–90.

Tassin, S. and Brucher, J. M. (1982), The mitochondrial disorders: pathogenesis and aetiological classification. *Neuropathol. Appl. Neurobiol.*, **8**, 251–63.

Tassin, S., Walter, G. F., Brucher, J. M. and Rousseau, J. J. (1980), Histochemical and ultrastructural analysis of the mitochondrial changes in a familial mitochondrial myopathy. *Neuropathol. Appl. Neurobiol.*, **6**, 337–47.

Tobin, W. E., Hijing, F., Porro, R. S. and Salzman, R. T. (1973), Muscle phosphofructokinase deficiency. *Arch. Neurol.*, **28**, 128–30.

Weller, R. O. and McArdle, B. (1971), Calcification within muscle fibres in the periodic paralyses. *Brain*, **94**, 263–72.

Willner, J., Di Mauro, S., Eastwood, A. *et al.* (1979), Muscle carnitine deficiency: genetic heterogeneity. *J. Neurol. Sci.*, **41**, 235–46.

9 Neurogenic disorders

The neurogenic disorders include diseases affecting anterior horn cells, nerve roots and peripheral nerves. In many of these there is involvement of neural pathways, other than the lower motor neuron. For example, in motor neuron disease there is almost always involvement of the upper motor neuron and in peripheral neuropathies sensory fibres are also involved. In this chapter only the changes seen in muscle biopsies will be described. A general account of the pathology of these disorders is given in other texts (e.g. Weller *et al.*, 1983). In many neurogenic disorders muscle biopsy is not indicated but in children muscle biopsy is useful in the diagnosis of spinal muscular atrophies and in adults, muscle biopsies are sometimes used in motor neuron disease when there is doubt about the diagnosis, particularly in patients with bulbar palsy without evident clinical involvement of the limbs. Sometimes muscle biopsies of adults with chronic neurogenic disorders are carried out to exclude polymyositis.

The blood CK level is usually normal in neurogenic disorders, but confusion may arise in chronic conditions, especially in Kugelberg–Welander disease, in chronic motor neuropathies, e.g. Charcot–Marie–Tooth disease, and in motor neuron disease, since in these neurogenic disorders the CK may be raised to as much as ten times above normal. This is often accompanied by the development of secondary changes of myopathic type (Schwartz *et al.*, 1976).

9.1 Spinal muscular atrophies

This group of disorders consists of a clinical syndrome of proximal muscular weakness and wasting of varying age of onset, progression and severity. They are inherited as autosomal recessive traits; sporadic cases are common. Several different forms are recognized, as listed in Table 9.1.

Weakness is often predominantly proximal especially in the late onset form, e.g. Type 3 spinal muscular atrophy and, although the disorder is

158

Table 9.1 Spinal muscular atrophies

	Age of onset	Outcome
Type 1 (Werdnig–Hoffmann disease)	Usually before 3 months	95% dead by age 18 months
Type 2 (Intermediate form)	6–12 months	Variable life expectancy, severe disability
Type 3 (Kugelberg–Welander disease)	2–15 years	Normal life expectancy, mild or moderate disability
Type 4 (Adult onset)	15–50 years	Mild disability

neurogenic in origin, the clinical features of the lower neuron lesion may be difficult to recognize. For example, fasciculation is often not present at rest. As a result these disorders are easily mistaken for myopathies and the finding of neurogenic change in the muscle biopsy may be unexpected.

9.1.1 Muscle biopsy

The pathological features differ in the various forms of spinal muscular atrophy, probably because of the effects of immaturity of the neuro-muscular system in the Type 1 and Type 2 forms.

In *Werdnig–Hoffmann disease* (Type 1 spinal muscular atrophy) the characteristic feature is the presence of large groups of small rounded atrophic fibres, which may encompass the whole fascicle. In addition, hypertrophied fibres, often three or four times normal size, are found intermingled with the atrophic fibres, and interfascicular fibrosis may be prominent (Fig. 9.1a, b). The rounded atrophic fibres may be of either fibre type, and may show fibre-type grouping of variable degree. The hypertrophied fibres are usually Type 1 fibres in ATPase preparations (Fig. 9.1c) but they show variable NADH reactivity suggesting that they have mixed histochemical characteristics. Other structures, for example nerves, blood vessels and muscle spindles, appear normal. Indeed, muscle spindles may appear unusually prominent because they are relatively resistant to denervation atrophy and thus are relatively preserved amidst the sheets of atrophic fibres so characteristic of the disease. Motor end-plates appear atrophic, and the terminal axons beaded and tortuous.

Fig. 9.1 Werdnig–Hoffmann disease. (a) × 140; HE. Fibrosis and loss of muscle fibres with hypertrophy of some of the remaining fibres are the major features. There are many tiny (<10μm) round fibres. (b) × 140; ATPase, pH 9.5. Perimysial thickening, loss of muscle fibres, and hypertrophy of both fibre types are prominent. There are many small rounded fibres and the distribution of atrophic and hypertrophied fibres is similar in the three fascicles illustrated. Fibre-type grouping is not a feature. (c) × 350; ATPase, pH 4.5. The hypertrophied fibres are darkly reactive Type 1 fibres. (d) × 140; HE. In this biopsy from an infant aged 2 weeks, fibre hypertrophy is not prominent although there are many areas of very small rounded fibres. (e) × 140; ATPase, pH 4.5. There is no fibre-type grouping, and fibrosis is not a feature. A few larger fibres are darkly reactive, but most fibres are atrophic.

The abnormality in the muscle biopsy in Type 1 spinal muscular atrophy varies according to the duration of the disease and the muscle biopsied. In particular, hypertrophied fibres may be absent, or less prominent, in biopsies taken in the first few weeks of life (Fig. 9.1d, e), but may appear a few months later (Dubowitz, 1978). The origin of these hypertrophied fibres thus relates to developmental factors, possibly to work hypertrophy, as muscles are used during development, the few remaining fibres being required to carry out normal tasks. In addition, spontaneous EMG activity has been recorded in this disease and this may be a factor leading to hypertrophy (see Swash and Schwartz, 1981). The atrophic fibres resemble immature, fetal muscle fibres in their histochemical and ultrastructural features and thus may represent maturational arrest, occurring as a result of denervation during fetal development (Hausmanowa-Petrusiewicz *et al.*, 1980).

Intermediate spinal muscular atrophy (Type 2) is uncommon. The muscle biopsy resembles that of Werdnig–Hoffmann disease, but fibre-type grouping is more prominent, including groups of small atrophic fibres, fibres of normal size and hypertrophied fibres (Fig. 9.2). Separate fascicles vary greatly in the degree of abnormality. Angulated fibres, characteristic of denervation in mature muscle are not found in Type 2 or Type 1 spinal muscular atrophy. The severity of the changes in the muscle biopsy in

(a)

Fig. 9.2 Intermediate (Type 2) spinal muscular atrophy. Child aged 6 years. (a) ×
380; HE. There are sheets of small rounded fibres of slightly varying size
occupying several fascicles: a nearby fascicle consists of larger fibres. The
perimysium is thickened. (b) × 380; ATPase, pH 4.5. The small fibres vary in
histochemical type and size. (c) × 380; ATPase, pH 4.5. The demarcation between
the small and the larger fibres is not necessarily abrupt or at a fascicular boundary.

Type 2 spinal muscular atrophy is not a reliable indicator of prognosis (Dubowitz and Brooke, 1973). In some biopsies in this condition, especially in older children who have entered a clinically stable phase of the disease, increased central nucleation and fibre splitting, indicative of secondary myopathic change may occur but this is usually mild. Sometimes core fibres and target fibres may occur.

Kugelberg–Welander disease (Type 3 spinal muscular atrophy) is the commonest form of this group of disorders. It may be clinically indistinguishable from proximal myopathy or limb–girdle muscular dystrophy and muscle biopsies often show prominent myopathic abnormalities, especially in older patients. These myopathic changes consist of degenerative and regenerative changes in individual fibres, muscle fibre splitting, hypertrophy and atrophy of fibres leading to abnormal variation in fibre size, central nucleation and endomysial and interfascicular fibrosis. Indeed, in HE preparations (Fig. 9.3) whether of formalin-fixed or frozen material, the biopsy may show such marked myopathic change, that the presence of the primary underlying neurogenic disorder may be missed. Enzyme histochemical studies, however, are diagnostic, since they reveal fibre-type grouping (Fig. 9.4). The groups consist of small groups of fibres of either histochemical type. The fibres in these groups are usually of normal size. In some biopsies some fascicles contain small, pointed, NADH-dark, atrophic fibres, whereas adjoining fascicles consist of fibres of normal size, arranged in the pattern of fibre-type grouping. The presence of these denervated atrophic fibres indicates failure of compensatory reinnervation, that is ineffective collateral sprouting, whereas the fibre-type groups represent effective reinnervation from collateral sprouting. The former may indicate that the disease is likely to be progressive. In many biopsies very large fibres, up to 150 μm diameter, may be seen. These are thought to result from work hypertrophy (Swash and Schwartz, 1977), and are particularly likely to show fibre splitting if examined in serial transverse sections.

Small, rounded atrophic fibres, similar to those found in Werdnig–Hoffmann disease, may also be found in Type 3 spinal muscular atrophy, suggesting that this disorder may also begin in infancy, although clinical presentation is delayed until childhood or adolescence.

Adult onset spinal muscular atrophy (Type 4) shows similar changes to those found in Kugelberg–Welander disease. Various other atypical forms have been reported. These include distal spinal muscular atrophy, patients with focal and non-progressive involvement of one limb, and others with a scapulo-peroneal pattern of weakness. These rare disorders show similar pathological features to those of Type 3 spinal muscular atrophy and thus form clinical syndromes without specific pathological features.

Fig. 9.3 Kugelberg–Welander disease (Type 3 spinal muscular atrophy). (a) ×
133; HE. There is markedly increased variation in fibre size and fibre splitting with
increased central nucleation and increased endomysial and perimysial connective
tissue. These are myopathic features, but the underlying neurogenic features are
apparent only in ATPase preparations. (b) × 560; HE. Fibre-splitting is associated
with central nucleation, or with regeneration as in the smaller granular fibre
(arrow).

Fig. 9.4   Kugelberg–Welander disease (Type 3 spinal muscular atrophy). × 140; ATPase, pH 4.3. There is type grouping of both Type 1 and Type 2 fibres, and the groups are very large, indicating effective reinnervation. Several clusters of small pointed denervated fibres are also present. The variability in fibre size within the fibre groups is apparent.

9.2 Motor neuron disease

This progressive and almost invariably fatal disease is usually readily diagnosed by clinical investigation. Presentation is usually as a mixed upper and lower motor neuron disorder, with weakness, atrophy, fasciculations and brisk tendon reflexes, but bulbar and lower motor neuron forms may occur and occasionally other atypical presentations such as primary ventilatory failure may lead to muscle biopsy. Asymmetrical involvement of the limbs is common and may be difficult to distinguish from the effects of vertebral spondylosis with root lesions. Death usually occurs in about 2 years from the onset of the disease, although some 15% of cases may survive for as long as 5 years.

9.2.1 Muscle biopsy

Three inter-related types of abnormality in this progressive disorder can be recognized (Table 9.2). These can be correlated with the stage of the disease, and the extent of compensatory reinnervation and other compensatory processes, e.g. fibre hypertrophy and fibre splitting.

Table 9.2 Pathological features in motor neuron disease

Denervation	Reinnervation	Other features
Small, angulated NADH-dark fibres	Fibre-type grouping (of normal-sized fibres)	Fibre hypertrophy (mainly Type 2 fibres)
Small group atrophy	Intermediate (Type 2C) fibres	Fibre splitting
Target fibres		Rare regenerating fibres

The most prominent abnormality is the presence of small angulated fibres, often found in small clusters (Fig. 9.5). These fibres may be of either histochemical type (Fig. 9.6), but react intensely in the NADH reaction (Fig. 9.7). This is the typical feature of *disseminated neurogenic atrophy*, a feature which may be the only abnormality in the earliest stages of the disease, for example, in a biopsy taken from a muscle of normal strength and bulk. In atrophic muscles, on the other hand, the disease process is more advanced. In these muscles *small group atrophy*, i.e. groups of atrophic fibres of the same histochemical type (Fig. 9.8) is found, and *fibre-type grouping*, i.e. groups of fibres of the same histochemical type and of normal size, is also a feature. The former is

Fig. 9.5 Motor neuron disease. × 140; HE. Post-mortem specimen. There are fibres of normal size, and clusters of smaller, pointed fibres (arrows) scattered through several fascicles.

Fig. 9.6 Motor neuron disease. × 140; ATPase, pH 4.3. The biopsy consists of Type 1 (dark), Type 2C (intermediate) and Type 2A and Type 2B (pale) fibres. There are a number of atrophic pointed (denervated) fibres of either histochemical type. Fibre-type grouping is not a feature of this case.

Fig. 9.7 Motor neuron disease. × 350; NADH. There are a number of pointed denervated fibres, two of which show targets. The latter are almost always restricted to Type 1 fibres.

Fig. 9.8 Motor neuron disease. × 140; ATPase, pH 4.3. Post-mortem specimen. Several small groups of atrophic Type 1, and Type 2 fibres are present. Fibre-type grouping is not prominent, but there is one area of Type 1 fibre grouping at the top of the field.

evidence of continuing denervation after compensatory reinnervation. The latter represents effective compensatory reinnervation by axonal sprouting. Target fibres are uncommon in motor neuron disease but may occur in the early stages (Figs 9.7, 9.8). They may be more prominent in cases with a rapidly progressive course. In motor neuron disease the groups of fibres in zones of fibre-type grouping are never as large (Fig. 9.9) as in the spinal muscular atrophies, or chronic motor neuropathies, in which whole fascicles may be of the same histochemical type (Fig. 9.10). There is no inflammatory cell response in the biopsy but, rarely, focal accumulations of lymphocytes may be noted. Fibre-type grouping, especially of Type 1 fibres, has been associated with a better prognosis, and the presence of clusters of atrophic fibres (Fig. 9.11) with a poor prognosis (Patten *et al.*, 1979), reflecting the relative preponderance of compensatory reinnervation by axonal sprouting. Axonal sprouting has been directly demonstrated (Cöers *et al.*, 1973; Wohlfart, 1957) by silver impregnation and by supravital methylene blue techniques, but such methods are of limited value in diagnosis. The peripheral nerves, like the ventral roots, show Wallerian degeneration and loss of motor axons.

In patients with a more slowly progressive course the muscle biopsy may show various additional abnormalities consistent with secondary myopathic change. Indeed Achari and Anderson (1974) found changes of

Fig. 9.9 Motor neuron disease. × 350; ATPase, pH 4.3. Type 1 fibre grouping is present, consisting of small groups (12–15 fibres), indicating that some collateral reinnervation has occurred.

Fig. 9.10 Old poliomyelitis. × 140; NADH. Two fascicles, each consisting of Type 1 or Type 2 fibre grouping. These groups are large, indicating effective collateral reinnervation. Note that the fibres are of uniform size.

Fig. 9.11   Motor neuron disease. × 140; ATPase, pH 9.5. Post-mortem specimen. One fascicle consists of almost uniformly atrophic pointed fibres. Since these fibres do not show fibre-type grouping, they demonstrate failure of effective reinnervation. Note the difference between this appearance and that of Type 2 spinal muscular atrophy shown in Fig. 9.2.

this type in 67% of a large series of cases. Fibre hypertrophy, mainly of Type 2 fibres (Fig. 9.12), is usually the most prominent such change, but this is not as marked as in more chronic neurogenic disorders, e.g. Type 3 spinal muscular atrophy. Fibre splitting, usually affecting these hypertrophied fibres, may also occur and less commonly isolated small basophilic regenerating fibres and slight endomysial fibrosis may occur. The blood CK is sometimes slightly raised in patients with these abnormalities (Schwartz et al., 1976).

In the final stages of the disease there is usually very advanced muscular wasting. Biopsies made at this time, or autopsy studies, show widespread grouped denervation atrophy, often with only a few zones of fibres of approximately normal size (Fig. 9.13). Fibrosis may be prominent in the interfascicular planes. The muscle spindles are denervated and appear enlarged (Fig. 9.11), although their intrafusal muscle fibres are atrophic (Swash and Fox, 1974).

The changes in the spinal cord and brain have been reviewed by Brownell et al (1970).

Fig. 9.12   Motor neuron disease. × 140; ATPase, pH 9.5. Post-mortem specimen. There is extensive fibre atrophy, with hypertrophy of many of the remaining functional Type 2 (dark) fibres. There are features of early secondary myopathic change consisting of rounding and increased variability in size of these Type 2 fibres. The muscle spindle appears prominent because of the loss of extrafusal skeletal muscle fibres.

9.3   Other disorders of anterior horn cells and ventral roots

In poliomyelitis and syringomyelia the abnormalities in the muscle biopsy differ from those found in motor neuron disease. The natural history of these disorders differs from that of motor neuron disease; in poliomyelitis the disorder is not progressive, so that compensatory reinnervation is well developed and fibre-type grouping prominent (Fig. 9.14). Furthermore, secondary myopathic changes may be very marked, even to the extent that a limited histological examination, for example, using only an HE preparation, may lead to a mistaken impression of an underlying myopathy (Drachman, *et al.*, 1967). Lesions of the ventral (motor) roots may also cause denervation and if recovery does not occur quickly there may be features of chronic partial denervation, i.e. grouped atrophy and fibre-type grouping, in a muscle biopsy (Fig. 9.15). Denervation changes also occur in Creutzfeld–Jakob disease and in patients with viral myelitis, especially that due to *Herpes zoster*.

Fig. 9.13 Motor neuron disease. × 140. Post-mortem specimen. (a) HE. There is marked fibre atrophy, although some fibres appear relatively normal. (b) ATPase, pH 9.5. The atrophic fibres are of both histochemical types. Fibre-type grouping is not prominent.

Fig. 9.14   Old poliomyelitis. × 140. ATPase, pH 9.5. Fibre-type grouping is very well developed, and the fibres are of more or less uniform size. The Type 1 fibres show slight hypertrophy. There are a few scattered atrophic denervated fibres, best seen in the Type 2 (dark fibre) group.

Fig. 9.15   Cervical root lesion. × 140; ATPase, pH 9.5. There is fibre-type grouping of Type 2 fibres (dark) to the left of the field. To the right there is Type 2 fibre atrophy with smaller groups of Type 2 fibres. The Type 1 fibres are of normal size and distribution.

9.4   Polyneuropathies

Muscle biopsies are rarely of diagnostic value in polyneuropathies since the diagnosis can usually be established by the clinical features, and by electromyographic tests, including nerve conduction studies. However, in some patients with slowly progressive motor neuropathies, without sensory involvement, diagnosis may be difficult and muscle biopsy may then be useful in that it will demonstrate the neurogenic disorder and indicate its chronicity and slow rate of progression. In acute neuropathies, e.g. Guillain–Barré polyradiculoneuropathy, muscle biopsy is not an investigation of choice but, again, it may be resorted to by the clinician when there is doubt about the diagnosis, usually in order to exclude acute polymyositis. In addition, muscle biopsies are occasionally carried out for similar reasons in patients with diabetic neuropathy and other acute or subacute neuropathies (see Table 1.1).

9.4.1   Chronic peripheral neuropathy

The majority of the chronic peripheral neuropathies, with prominent motor involvement, are of genetic origin (see Swash and Schwartz, 1981). The most common of these are the Types I and II forms of peroneal muscular atrophy (Charcot–Marie–Tooth disease). In the Type I disease the underlying cause is a demyelinating neuropathy in which the peripheral nerves are thickened due to reduplication of Schwannian cytoplasmic rings surrounding axons, the characteristic 'onion bulb' formations, with endoneurial fibrosis. In the Type II form the underlying abnormality is an axonal neuropathy, perhaps due to primary disease of the neuron itself. The nerve conduction velocity is very slowed in the Type I disorder, and the spinal fluid protein raised. In the Type II form, however, the nerve conduction velocity is only slightly slowed and the CSF protein is normal, or only slightly raised. The clinical features of the other forms of genetic neuropathy have been reviewed elsewhere (Dyck et al., 1975; Swash and Schwartz, 1981).

(a) *Muscle biopsy*. In weak, wasted distal muscles the typical features of denervation and reinnervation are seen. These include small, angulated, atrophic fibres, which may occur in clusters, with small groups of atrophic fibres of the same histochemical type. This is associated with large groups of fibres, of one histochemical type, often comprising a whole fascicle. Individual fibres within these large groups often vary in size. Hypertrophy of Type 1 fibres is prominent, and these fibres may measure more than 150 μm diameter. Central nucleation and fibre splitting are commonly found in such fibres and a few scattered basophilic regenerating fibres may be noted. The Type 2 fibres are often somewhat atrophic, in contrast to the Type 1 fibres, but these are also arranged in groups; fibre-type grouping is thus a feature both of Type 1 and Type 2 fibres. Target and targetoid fibres may occur. The myopathic features noted above are frequently very prominent and it is therefore essential to study biopsies of such patients with a suitable range of enzyme histochemical methods, since fibre-type grouping can only be recognized with these methods, and the diagnosis depends on this observation.

The muscle biopsy is similar in the Type I and Type II forms of the disease, despite the apparently differing underlying abnormality in the peripheral nervous system. Presumably, this indicates that axonal damage is a feature of both forms of Charcot–Marie–Tooth disease (Buchthal and Behse, 1977), although the primary abnormality in the Type I disorder affects the Schwann cells, rather than the axons. In the other genetically determined (Table 1.1) chronic neuropathies similar changes occur in the muscle, depending on the severity, rate of progression and duration of the motor component of the disorder. Muscle biopsies are rarely carried out in these disorders, but nerve biopsies may be useful in characterizing them, e.g. in amyloid neuropathy, leprosy and sulphatide lipidosis (metachromatic leucodystrophy).

9.4.2   Acute and subacute peripheral neuropathies

These disorders are principally characterized by denervation; reinnervation is not prominent since the disorder is of recent onset, or acute and self-limited as in Guillain–Barré syndrome.

(a) *Muscle biopsy.* The hallmark of these disorders is disseminated neurogenic atrophy with little or no grouped atrophy or fibre-type grouping. Small groups of atrophic fibres may be seen scattered in the biopsy. Both fibre types show atrophy. Hypertrophy is rare. Targets and targetoid fibres may be prominent, and atrophic, angulated fibres often show prominent pyknotic nuclei. The biopsy shows no more specific features and is of little value in characterizing the cause of the neuropathy.

In diabetic amyotrophy similar findings occur in the early stages. Tubular aggregates may be a feature of some cases (Chokroverty *et al.*, 1977). Later in the disease, fibre-type grouping may develop. In uraemic neuropathy, an example of a demyelinating neuropathy which is reversible with effective treatment, the muscle biopsy shows little or no abnormality.

Table 9.3 Histological features of neurogenic disorders

	Spinal Muscular Atrophy		Motor Neuron Disease		Neuropathies	
	Types I and II	*Types III and IV*	*Early*	*Late*	*Acute*	*Chronic*
Fibre size	Small round fibres Hypertrophied fibres (Type 1)	Small angular fibres Few small rounded fibres Prominent very hypertrophied fibres (Type 1)	Scattered small angular fibres	Small and large fibres	Scattered small angular fibres or normal	Small and large fibres
Small group atrophy		+	±	+		±
Large group atrophy		+		+		+
Fibre type grouping	+	++		+		++
Myopathic features		++		+		++

9.5   Mononeuropathies

Most mononeuropathies are due to nerve entrapment or external trauma to a nerve, and muscle biopsy is not indicated. However, in mononeuropathies associated with collagen vascular disease, e.g. polyarteritis nodosa and other forms of autoimmune or allergic vasculitis, such as Churg–Strauss syndrome, muscle biopsy is sometimes suggested as a useful investigation. Nonetheless, random biopsy of a proximal muscle almost invariably fails to substantiate the diagnosis in patients with polyarteritis, and muscle biopsy is probably not, therefore, worth attempting in such cases (Wallace *et al.*, 1958). If muscle biopsy is arranged in an attempt to establish a diagnosis of vasculitis, a large open biopsy should be taken and transverse sections taken at multiple levels in order to search for perivascular lymphocytic, plasma cell or eosinophil infiltrates, or fibrinoid necrosis. Formalin-fixed, paraffin-embedded tissue is more convenient for this purpose than frozen tissue, perhaps the only indication for this preparative technique remaining in muscle biopsy work. Rarely, features of inflammatory myopathy, and intrafascicular muscle infarction may be recognized in this disorder.

9.5.1   *Comparative features of muscle biopsy pathology in neurogenic disorders*

The various features of the major neurogenic disorders are summarized in Table 9.3.

References

Achari, A. N. and Anderson, M. S. (1974), Myopathic changes in amyotrophic lateral sclerosis. *Neurosurg (Minneap.)*, **24**, 477–81.
Brownell, B., Oppenheimer, D. R. and Hughes, J. T. (1970), The central nervous system in motor neuron disease. *J. Neurol. Neurosurg. Psychiatry*, **33**, 338–57.
Buchthal, F. and Behse, F. (1977), Peroneal muscular atrophy (PMA) and related disorders. 1. Clinical manifestation as related to biopsy findings, nerve conduction and electromyography. *Brain*, **100**, 41–6.
Chokroverty, S., Reyes, M. G., Rubino, F. A. and Tonaki, H. (1977), The syndrome of diabetic amyotrophy. *Ann. Neurol.*, **2**, 181–94.
Coërs, C., Telerman-Toppet, N. and Gerard, J-M. (1973), Terminal innervation ratio in neurosmuscular disease: disorders of lower motor neuron, peripheral nerve and muscle. *Arch. Neurol.*, **29**, 215–22.
Drachman, D. B., Murphy, J. R. N., Nigam, M. P. and Hills, J. R. (1967), 'Myopathic' changes in chronically denervated muscle. *Arch. Neurol.*, **16**, 14–24.
Dubowitz, V. (1978), *Muscle Disorders in Childhood*, W. B. Saunders, London.
Dubowitz, V. and Brooke, M. H. (1973), *Muscle Biopsy – A Modern Approach*, W. B. Saunders, London.
Dyck, P. J., Thomas, P. K. and Lambert, E. M. (1975), *Peripheral Neuropathy*, Vols 1 and 2, Saunders, Philadelphia.

Hausmanowa-Petrusiewicz, I., Fidzianska, A., Niebros-Dobrosz, I. and Strugal-ska, M. H. (1980), Is Kugelberg-Welander spinal muscular atrophy a fetal defect? *Muscle Nerve*, **3**, 389–402.

Patten, B. M., Zito, G. and Horati, Y. (1979), Histologic findings in motor neuron disease. *Arch. Neurol.*, **36**, 560–4.

Schwartz, M. S., Sargeant, M. K. and Swash, M. (1976), Longitudinal fibre splitting in neurogenic muscular disorders – its relation to the pathogenesis of myopathic change. *Brain*, **99**, 617–36.

Swash, M. and Fox, K. P. (1974), The pathology of the human muscle spindle: effect of denervation. *J. Neurol. Sci.* **22**, 1–24.

Swash, M. and Schwartz, M. S. (1977), Implications of longitudinal muscle fibre splitting in neurogenic and myopathic disorders. *J. Neurol. Nuerosurg. Psychiatry*, **40**, 1152–9.

Swash, M. and Schwartz, M. S. (1981), *Neuromuscular Diseases: A Practical Approach to Diagnosis and Mangement*, Springer-Verlag, Berlin, Heidelberg, New York.

Wallace, S. L., Lattis, R. and Ragan, C. (1958), Diagnostic significance of the muscle biopsy. *Am. J. Med.*, **25**, 600–10.

Weller, R. O., Swash, M., McLellan, D. L. and Scholtz, C. (1983), *Clinical Neuropathology*, Springer-Verlag, Heidelberg, Berlin, New York.

Wohlfart, G. (1957), Collateral regeneration from residual motor nerve fibres in amyotrophic lateral sclerosis. *Neurology (Minneap.)*, **7**, 124–34.

10 Tumours of striated muscle, and related disorders

Tumours in striated muscle are uncommon. Most are primary tumours but not all of these represent primary tumours of muscle cells since neoplasms may arise in other tissues in muscle, for example, fibrous tissue, blood vessels, fat and nerve fibres. In addition neoplasms arising in contiguous structures such as bone or tendon, may invade muscle. Metastases in muscle are rarely clinically apparent, and thus unlikely to present for biopsy. However, microscopic metastases are probably relatively common, occurring in 16% of one series of patients with malignant disease studied at autopsy (Pearson, 1959). Recently, CT scanning has been shown to be useful in the clinical assessment of soft tissue tumours, and in the detection of metastases (Golding and Husband, 1982).

Metastatic tumours in muscle are more commonly complications of lymphomas than carcinomas. Skeletal muscles are most likely to be involved by cancer from other sites by contiguous extension of the tumour from neighbouring structures. Once having invaded the muscle, spread may occur along fascial planes or even along the sarcolemmal tubes of the muscle fibres themselves (Slatkin and Pearson, 1976). The muscle may be further damaged by the effects of compression by the tumour on the muscle, on its nerve supply, or on its blood vessels, causing infarction, haemorrhage, oedema and thus regenerative changes, or features of denervation in the muscle at the margins of the tumour.

10.1 Primary tumours arising in muscle

A classification of primary tumours arising in muscle is given in Table 10.1. Many of these lesions are particularly uncommon in limb muscles. Other mass lesions, sometimes referred to as pseudotumours, consisting of inflammatory or xanthomatous change, may also present as muscle tumours (Table 10.2).

180

Table 10.1 Primary tumours arising in muscle

Tumours of muscle tissue
  Benign: rhabdomyoma
  Malignant: rhabdomyosarcoma
                embryonal
                alveolar
                pleomorphic

Tumours of fibrous tissue
  Benign: tumour-like disorders
                nodular pseudosarcomatous fasciitis (or proliferative fasciitis)
                desmoid tumours
                    abdominal wall
                    extrabdominal
                other forms of fibromatosis (see Table 10.3)
  Malignant: fibrosarcoma

Tumours of fat
  Benign: Intramuscular lipoma
                hibernoma
  Malignant: liposarcoma

Tumours of blood vessels
  Benign: intramuscular haemangioma
                systemic haemangiomatosis
                haemangio-pericytoma
  Malignant: haemangio-pericytoma
                angiosarcoma

Other tumours that may arise in muscle
  Benign: myxoma
                granular cell myoblastoma
                Schwannomas (of peripheral nerve)
  Malignant: alveolar soft part sarcoma
                malignant fibrous histiocytoma
                synovial sarcoma

Table 10.2 Muscle masses that mimic tumours (pseudotumours)

Haematoma

Inflammatory lesions
    focal myositis
    myositis ossificans
    sarcoidosis

Xanthomas

10.1.1 Rhabdomyoma

This is an exceedingly rare benign tumour of striated muscle, predominantly affecting young men aged 25–40 years and almost invariably found in the head and neck region. The tumour consists of polygonal cells, frequently containing PAS-positive vacuoles (glycogen). These cells show cross-striations with PTAH stains and may resemble those found in cardiac rhabdomyomas.

10.1.2 Rhabdomyosarcoma

This malignant tumour represents 10–20% of all sarcomas of soft tissue origin, and is the most common soft tissue sarcoma of childhood. Three histological types, embryonal, alveolar and pleomorphic, are recognized, and these can be correlated with the site of origin of the tumour. Botryoid features, i.e. an appearance resembling bunches of grapes, occur in the embryonal type. The embryonal type is commonest in children under 10 years of age, the alveolar variety occurs in young adults (Enzinger and Shiraki, 1969) and the pleomorphic type is commonest in the 5th decade. Embryonal rhabdomyosarcomas usually arise in orbits, nasopharynx, lower urogenital tract and bile ducts. The alveolar and pleomorphic types arise in the limb muscles, and to a lesser extent in the trunk. The thigh is the commonest site of origin of pleomorphic rhabdomyosarcomas but alveolar tumours arise equally frequently in arms, legs and trunk.

The tumour (Fig. 10.1) consists of pink tissue of variable consistency. Microscopic examination shows a variety of different types of tumour cells, with varying patterns of cellular organization so that vascular, myxoid, alveolar or solid forms may coexist in the same tumour. Fibrosed areas may be a feature. The predominant cell type is the embryonal rhabdomyoblast; when undifferentiated this is a small round or oval cell with prominent vesicular nuclei. Spindle-shaped cells, which may show cross-striation in HE and PTAH, are found in more differentiated areas of the tumour (Fig. 10.2). Myofibrils can more easily be identified in ATPase and NADH preparations of frozen material (Sarnat, et al., 1979). An alveolar arrangement is common and, when prominent, forms the basis for the subclassification of these tumours. Multinucleated giant cells are common in the alveolar form. Mitoses are found in all three types but

Fig. 10.1   × 171; HE. Embryonal rhabdomyosarcoma. A tumour from a boy aged 6 years showing sheets of undifferentiated cells.
Fig. 10.2   × 617; HE. Embryonal rhabdomyosarcoma. Same case as Fig. 10.1, photographed with partial crossed polaroids to show cross striations in spindle-shaped cells. The nuclei vary in shape. Some are small and round, others are elongated, or sometimes large and irregular.

are commonest in the embryonal form. Bizarre, multinucleated cells, vacuolated cells and cells containing large nucleoli are frequently found. Ultrastructural studies reveal myofibrils in an active cytoplasm; the appearances resemble those of developing myoblasts. Rhabdomyosarcomas metastasise widely through the blood stream, and the metastases resemble the primary neoplasm.

10.2   Tumours and tumour-like disorders of fibrous tissue

These are broadly classified as benign; *fibromatoses*, and malignant; *fibrosarcomas* (Table 10.1). The latter are uncommon.

10.2.1   Fibromatoses

The term *fibromatosis* has been used to describe an infiltrating fibroblastic proliferation without inflammation or features of neoplasia. They may be diffuse or multifocal, or present as localized nodules at any site and in patients of any age. Affected tissues are replaced or infiltrated by well-differentiated fibroblasts. Mitotic figures are not a feature. These lesions do not metastasise. However, their cellularity may lead to difficulty in making a distinction from fibrosarcomas. Mackenzie (1972) has attempted an overall classification of these lesions (Table 10.3).

Of the disorders listed in Table 10.3, proliferative myositis and fasciitis, desmoid tumours, fibrous hamartoma of infancy, juvenile fibromatosis and fibromatosis colli affect muscle, but all these lesions are rare.

Desmoid tumours characteristically present as a superficial painless

Table 10.3 Fibromatoses (after Mackenzie, 1972)

Congenital and juvenile fibromatoses
  Fibrous hamartoma of infancy
  Fibromatosis colli
  Infantile and juvenile fibromatoses
  Juvenile aponeurotic fibroma
  Congenital generalized fibromatosis

Miscellaneous fibromatoses
  Palmar and plantar fibromatosis (Dupuytren's contracture)
  Mesenteric fibromatosis
  Musculo-aponeurotic fibromatosis (Desmoid tumours)
  Generalized multifocal fibromatosis
  Hereditary gingival fibromatosis
  Proliferative fasciitis (Chung and Enzinger, 1975)
  Proliferative myositis (Enzinger and Dulcey, 1967)
  ?Fibrous dysplasia of bone

lump related to tendons or to the abdominal wall musculature. The mass consists of whorls of small fibroblasts in a collagenous stroma. *Proliferative myositis* consists of a poorly demarcated, scar-like, indurated mass in muscle usually occurring in a patient older than 45 years. Histologically there are two main features. There is fibroblastic proliferation, involving the epimysium and endomysium, with large basophilic giant cells. The cellular elements are intermixed with collagen and mucoid material (Enzinger and Dulcey, 1967). *Proliferative fasciitis* is related to proliferative myositis. This lesion consists of a poorly demarcated mass in the subcutaneous tissue superficial to muscle and probably arising from the superficial fascia. The characteristic features consist of a mixture of large basophilic giant cells and fibroblast-like spindle cells surrounded by a myxoid matrix (Chung and Enzinger, 1975).

10.2.2 Fibrosarcoma

This malignant tumour may arise at any site, but occurs most commonly in the thigh musculature. The mean age of onset is in the fifth decade and the duration of survival can be related to the histological grade of malignancy of the tumour. About 50% of cases survive five years from diagnosis (Pritchard *et al.*, 1974). The tumour is usually nodular and may appear encapsulated; nevertheless metastases occur through the blood stream to lung, liver and bone in about 60% of cases. Lymphatic metastases are rare.

It is difficult to assess the behaviour of the tumour by histological examination. Some tumours consist of a large amount of collagen, containing fibroblasts of varying size and shape arranged in interlaced bands. In others there is less collagen, the tumour is more cellular, and the cells are spindle shaped without evidence of differentiation. Mitotic figures are frequent. In some cases the fibroblastic cells are arranged in a herring-bone pattern; this appearance leads to difficulty in distinguishing this tumour from malignant fibrous histiocytoma.

10.3 Tumours of fat

Lipomas may arise in any site and intramuscular lipomas are not uncommon. As a rule the cells in the lipoma are well differentiated and this serves to distinguish this benign tumour from *liposarcoma*. However, an atypical appearance has been described in intramuscular lipomas (Evans *et al.*, 1979). Liposarcoma may sometimes occur in or involve muscle. *Hibernoma* is a rare tumour of brown fat consisting of granular or vacuolated acidophilic cells; the tumour usually presents in the shoulder or neck.

10.4 Tumours of blood vessels

Intramuscular haemangioma may be capillary, cavernous or arteriovenous. These tumours may diffusely infiltrate skeletal muscle, and are found chiefly in young adults. They are histologically and clinically benign. *Haemangiopericytoma* may be benign or malignant. This tumour usually presents as a painless, well circumscribed mass in the thigh or pelvis of adults. Most are of homogeneous appearance but with small areas of haemorrhage, necrosis or cystic degeneration. Rarely massive haemorrhage may occur. The tumour consists of tightly packed, uniform round, oval or spindle-shaped cells surrounding thin-walled vascular spaces. It may be difficult to distinguish this tumour from other well-vascularized mesenchymal tumours, such as synovial sarcoma, and malignant fibroxanthoma. Haematogenous metastases occur in about 15% of malignant haemangiopericytoma, in which mitotic figures are an important feature. In general the prognosis is related to the size of the tumour (Enzinger and Smith, 1976).

10.5 Other tumours that may arise in muscle

10.5.1 Benign tumours

Myxomas are usually benign, and often arise in thigh and shoulder muscle. They may readily be recognized by the mucoid material, consisting largely of hyaluronic acid, in which small round or spindle-shaped cells and reticulin and collagen fibrils can be seen. Utrastructural studies suggest that myxomas in muscle are derived from Schwann cells. *Granular cell tumour* (myoblastoma) is a benign tumour usually arising in subcutaneous or submucous tissue, especially the tongue, but sometimes occurring in skeletal muscle. It consists of large rounded or spindle cells, which are granular and acidophilic and which contain small dark nuclei (Fig. 10.3). This tumour only rarely shows malignant change. *Schwannomas* may also present within muscle from their site of origin on peripheral nerves; they may sometimes be malignant (Ghosh *et al.*, 1973).

Fig. 10.3 × 171; HE. Granular cell myoblastoma. Nodule from the thigh of a woman aged 29 years. Groups of large eosinophilic granular cells with small regular nuclei are separated by loose collagen.
Fig. 10.4 × 171; HE. Alveolar soft part sarcoma. Tumour from the thigh of a girl aged 16 years. The alveolar arrangement of the tumour is seen with fine vascular channels separating groups of cells, some of which have broken down centrally.

Fig. 10.7 × 617; HE. Malignant fibrous histiocytoma. Same case as Fig. 10.3 demonstrating cellular pleomorphism and bizarre giant cells.

10.5.2   Malignant tumours

(a) *Alveolar soft part sarcoma.* This tumour usually arises in the limbs, especially in the thigh. The tumour is commoner in women than in men, and usually presents in the third or fourth decade (Hajdu, 1979). The tumour infiltrates soft tissues and metastasises widely. It consists of polygonal, coarsely granular cells arranged in an alveolar pattern (Fig. 10.4) or in compact groups. These cells have an eosinophilic cytoplasm (Fig. 10.5) which stains light brown in trichrome and PTAH stains; the granules are PAS positive and diastase resistant. Endothelial cell-lined,

---

Fig. 10.5 × 617; HE. Alveolar soft part sarcoma. High magnification of the tumour seen in Fig. 10.4 showing the eosinophilic granular appearance of the better preserved cells at the periphery of the clumps.

Fig. 10.6 × 171; HE. Malignant fibrous histiocytoma. A tumour from the deep fascia of a man aged 68. The cartwheel or storiform pattern is seen. There is much cellular pleomorphism, including giant cells.

thin vascular channels and septa are prominent. Mitotic figures are usually present. The five-year survival is 60% (Lieberman *et al.*, 1966).

(b) *Malignant fibrous histiocytoma*. This is a deep-seated malignant neoplasm probably of histiocytic origin although two cell lines, histiocytic and mesenchymal, occur in most examples of this tumour. It has sometimes been termed malignant fibroxanthoma. The peak incidence is in the seventh decade and it is rare under the age of 40 years. The thigh and buttock are the most common sites of origin. Metastases occur in about 40% of cases. It is the most common soft tissue sarcoma of late adult life.

The tumour is multilobulated and fleshy. Microscopically it has a highly variable appearance. Three patterns have been recognized; cartwheel (storiform) (Fig. 10.6), pleomorphic (Fig. 10.7) and fascicular. Inflammatory cells are common, set in a collagenous stroma. This tumour has been reviewed by Weiss and Enzinger (1978).

(c) *Synovial sarcoma*. This malignant tumour presents most commonly in the region of the knee, foot and ankle joints. It may involve the nearby muscles by contiguity. Two features are characteristic of this tumour; a spindle cell fibrosarcoma-like element and a pseudoepithelial element. Well-differentiated tumours carry a better prognosis, but the five-year survival is only about 50%. The tumour may occur at any age (Mackenzie, 1966).

In conclusion, although the diagnosis of tumours arising in muscle is often difficult it is particularly important to recognize those tumours whose biological behaviour is malignant since the treatment of choice is wide surgical excision. Radiotherapy has little to offer in the management of malignancies arising in muscle. Benign lesions simply require local excision.

References

Chung, E. B. and Enzinger, F. M. (1975), Proliferative fasciitis. *Cancer*, **36**, 1450–8.
Enzinger, F. M. and Dulcey, F. (1967), Proliferative myositis: a report of 33 cases. *Cancer*, **20**, 2213–23.
Enzinger, F. M. and Shiraki, M. (1969), Alveolar rhabdomyosarcoma: an analysis of 110 cases. *Cancer*, **24**, 18–31.
Enzinger, F. M. and Smith, B. H. (1976), Haemangiopericytoma: an analysis of 106 cases. *Hum. Pathol.*, **7**, 61–82.
Evans, H. L., Soule, E. H. and Winkelmann, R. K. (1979), Atypical lipoma, atypical intramuscular lipoma and well differentiated retroperitoneal liposarcoma. *Cancer*, **43**, 574–84.
Ghosh, B. D., Ghosh, L., Huvos, A. G. and Fartner, J. G. (1973), Malignant schwannoma: a clinico-pathologic study. *Cancer*, **31**, 184–90.
Golding, S. J. and Husband, J. E. (1982), Radiology of soft tissue sarcoma: discussion paper. *J. R. Soc. Med.*, **75**, 729–35.

Hajdu, S. I. (1979), *Pathology of Soft Tissue Tumour*, Leo & Febiger, Philadelphia, pp. 352–3.

Lieberman, P. H., Foote, F. W., Stewart, F. W. and Berg, J. W. (1966), Alveolar soft part sarcoma. *JAMA*, **198**, 1047–51.

Mackenzie, D. H. (1966), Synovial sarcoma: a review of 58 cases. *Cancer*, **19**, 169–80.

Mackenzie, D. H. (1972) The fibromatoses: a clinicopathological concept. *Br. Med. J.*, **4**, 277–81.

Pearson, C. M. (1959), Incidence and type of pathologic alterations observed in muscle in a routine autopsy survey. *Neurology (Minneap.)*, **9**, 757–66.

Pritchard, D. J., Soule, E. H., Taylor, W. F. and Ivins, J. C. (1974), Fibrosarcoma: a clinicopathologic and statistical study of 199 tumors of the soft tissue of extremities and trunk. *Cancer*, **33**, 888–97.

Sarnat, H., de Mello, D. E. and Siddiqui, S. Y. (1979), Diagnostic value of histochemistry in embryonal rhabdomyosarcoma. *Am. J. Surg. Pathol.* **3**, 177–83.

Slatkin, D. N. and Pearson, J. (1976), Intramyofiber metastases in skeletal muscle. *Hum. Pathol.*, **7**, 347–9.

Weiss, S. W. and Enzinger, F. M. (1978), Malignant fibrous histiocytoma, an analysis of 200 cases. *Cancer*, **41**, 2250–66.

11 Interpretation of the muscle biopsy

Although enzyme histochemical techniques are needed to establish an accurate diagnosis in many neuromuscular disorders, some diagnoses can be established without them by using formalin-fixed, paraffin-embedded material stained with HE alone or with additional slides prepared by the PAS, PTAH or van Giesen techniques. For example, typical cases of untreated polymyositis in which inflammation is prominent pose no difficulty in diagnosis, and there is similarly no difficulty in recognizing typical examples of Duchenne muscular dystrophy or muscle tumours. However, less advanced or less typical cases are more difficult to recognize without the range of techniques available in enzyme histochemistry and electron microscopy and in some disorders, e.g. chronic neurogenic disorders, the diagnosis can easily be missed without these methods.

11.1 Is the biopsy abnormal?

In examining a muscle biopsy it is important, first of all, to establish whether or not the biopsy is abnormal. Even gross examination of the fresh specimen is sometimes sufficient to reveal the presence of increased amounts of fat, or of fibrous tissue, and simple naked-eye examination of the slides will also reveal such gross changes without recourse to microscopy. However, it is not always so easy to decide whether a biopsy is abnormal. For example, biopsies taken from muscles that are only mildly affected, or are clinically unaffected, may show very slight abnormalities, for example, changes in fibre size, or increased central nucleation. Such abnormalities may not themselves be significant since they may occur in normal individuals, especially after excessive physical training or injury to muscle. Caution is particularly important when studies of relatives are undertaken in families with inherited muscular dystrophy.

192

11 Myopathic or neurogenic?

In abnormal muscles a broad distinction between a myopathic or neurogenic process can usually be made and this is of great importance in subsequent decisions as to the specific abnormality. It may not be possible to make a more specific diagnosis but the distinction is important to the clinician concerned with establishing the diagnosis from the whole database available from other clinical and investigative methods. In some disorders, especially polymyositis and some chronic neurogenic disorders, a mixture of features of these two broad divisions of muscle abnormalities may be present, and these may therefore pose special difficulties in diagnosis. The major histological features of myopathic and neurogenic disorders are shown in Table 11.1, in the order of their diagnostic specificity. All of these abnormalities will not be found in any

Table 11.1 The histological features of myopathic and neurogenic disorders (arranged in order of their diagnostic importance and specificity)

Myopathic	Neurogenic
Necrosis and regeneration of individual muscle fibres	Fibre-type grouping
	Grouped neurogenic atrophy
Increased variability in fibre size	
	Disseminated neurogenic (small group) atrophy
Rounded fibres	
	Scattered single atrophic fibres
Fibrosis	
	Target or core-targetoid fibres
Architectural changes in fibres	
	Secondary myopathic features in chronic neurogenic disorders (see Table 4.13)
Various specific morphological abnormalities (see Table 11.3)	
Type 1 fibre predominance	Type 1 fibre hypertrophy
Type 2 fibre atrophy	Type 2 fibre predominance
Central nucleation	
Perifascicular atrophy and inflammatory cell infiltrates in polymyositis	
Fibre-type grouping uncommon except in polymyositis	

individual biopsy, or even necessarily in a particular disorder. For example, in an acute neurogenic disorder target fibres and scattered atrophic, pointed fibres may be prominent, but fibre-type grouping and grouped neurogenic atrophy will probably not be present since insufficient time will have elapsed to allow reinnervation by axonal sprouting and then denervation of the resulting groups of reinnervated muscle fibres. Similarly, in a metabolic myopathy fibre necrosis and regeneration may be rare, but other more specific features such as ragged-red fibres or abnormalities in muscle glycogen and fat may be prominent. Central nucleation is often found in myopathic disorders, and in these disorders it may be a feature of fibres of more or less normal size. It also occurs, however, in chronic neurogenic disorders, in which it is found mainly in hypertrophied fibres and is a feature associated with fibre splitting. Fibrosis is far more common in myopathic than in neurogenic disorders but fatty infiltration may occur in the late stages of either group of neuromuscular diseases. In polymyositis, particularly chronic polymyositis, myopathic features may coexist with inflammatory cell infiltrates and with fibre-type grouping. The latter is not usually prominent, but consists of small groups of fibres of the same histochemical type.

In practice, many biopsies show only minimal abnormalities, the changes shown in Table 11.1 being more typical of more advanced disease. In *mild myopathic disorders* increased central nucleation, rounded fibres, slight architectural changes in some fibres, usually Type 1 fibres, and Type 2 fibre atrophy may be the main abnormalities. Regenerating fibres may not be prominent. In *mild neurogenic disorders* small pointed denervated fibres may be seen scattered or isolated in the biopsy with little other abnormality.

11.3   Specific morphological changes in myopathies

The common histological features of myopathies are found developed to varying degrees in biopsies of different disorders, and the particular pattern of abnormality in the biopsy is important in diagnosis. The significance of these abnormalities is indicated in Table 11.2. Various specific morphological abnormalities occur in muscle fibres in different disorders and these are of particular importance in diagnosis, although some, for example rod bodies, are often found as a non-specific feature in muscle biopsies. Only when they are present as the major abnormality can they confidently be regarded as a pathognomonic feature. These abnormalities, many of which are uncommon, are discussed in relation to their diagnostic significance below.

Table 11.2 Significance of common abnormalities in muscle biopsies

Increased central nucleation
    Common in myopathies
    Chains of central nuclei in *myotonic dystrophy*
    Plump, enlarged, vesicular central nuclei in regenerating fibres
    Central nucleation in hypertrophied fibres, especially Type 1 fibres in *chronic neurogenic disorders* and *chronic* polymyositis

Necrotic fibres
    Any active myopathy, particularly polymyositis
    Muscular dystrophies
    Toxic myopathies

Ghost fibres
    A necrotic fibre consisting of the basal lamina, with only pale remnants of sarcoplasm remaining

Basophilic regenerating fibres
    Polymyositis
    Muscular dystrophies
    Recovery after acute muscle fibre necrosis in toxic myopathies

Type 1 fibre predominance
    Metabolic myopathies
    Duchenne muscular dystrophy
    Limb-girdle muscular dystrophy

Perifascicular atrophy
    Childhood-type dermatomyositis

Fibrosis
    Duchenne muscular dystrophy, even at an early stage
    Other muscular dystrophies
    Chronic polymyositis
    Some chronic neurogenic disorders

Adipose tissue in muscle
    Late stage of neurogenic or myopathic disorders
    Interfascicular fat common in Duchenne dystrophy

Hyaline fibres
    Common in Duchenne dystrophy, but occasionally a feature of limb-girdle dystrophy

11.4   Significance of some morphological abnormalities in muscle fibres

Increased neutral fat droplets: usually in Type 1 fibres, especially a feature of carnitine deficiency. May occur also in Type 1 fibres in steroid myopathy, alcoholic myopathy and in scattered single fibres in Duchenne muscular dystrophy. Fibres containing increased numbers of lipid droplets are also a feature of mitochondrial myopathies, but these fibres also contain excessive glycogen.

Ragged-red fibres: a feature of mitochondrial myopathies and of other uncharacterized myopathies, associated with involvement of ocular muscles, in which ragged-red fibres are the major abnormality. Ragged-red fibres also occur, in small numbers, in other diseases, e.g. polymyositis, limb–girdle myopathies, but other changes are more prominent in these cases. Carnitine deficiency is also associated with ragged-red fibres.

Increased glycogen (PAS-positive material, digestible with diastase): found in the muscle glycogenoses, especially McArdle's disease in which the glycogen appears diffusely through the sarcoplasm. PAS-positive vacuoles are prominent in acid maltase and debranching enzyme deficiency. In the former these vacuoles are lysosomal, and show a positive reaction for acid phosphatase. The glycogen content of muscle fibres is also increased in mitochondrial myopathies.

Rod bodies: when found in subsarcolemmal location, and when very numerous, especially in children, rod bodies suggest nemaline (rod body) myopathy. They also occur in central core disease. Rod bodies are also found in denervation, polymyositis, schizophrenia and after tenotomy, and similar abnormalities occur in degenerate myofilaments in many other neuromuscular disorders as a non-specific phenomenon. In these instances the rod bodies are not usually so strikingly located in the subsarcolemmal region as in nemaline myopathy itself.

Central cores: a cardinal feature of central core disease, and in malignant hyperpyrexia. Cores, core-targetoid and target fibres may be difficult to differentiate, and may represent different stages of the same pathological process. *Multicores* (minicores) and *focal loss of cross-striations* may also be recognized (see Chapter 7).

Tubular aggregates: a non-specific abnormality of Type 2B fibres, reported in myotonic dystrophy, hypokalaemic and hyperkalaemic periodic paralysis and in diabetic amyotrophy.

Vacuoles: may contain fat, or glycogen, or represent fluid-filled membrane-bound spaces in the muscle fibres. Glycogen-filled vacuoles occur in acid maltase and debrancher enzyme deficiency, and fluid-filled vacuoles, derived from the tubular system of the muscle fibres are a feature of hypokalaemic myopathies. In periodic paralysis these vacuoles contain a faintly PAS-positive, diastase-resistant material. Lipid-filled vacuoles occur in lipid storage myopathies, e.g. carnitine deficiency, in alcoholic myopathy and in steroid myopathy. Other forms of storage material have been recognized in muscle tissue, but these disorders do not cause muscular weakness and are not usually diagnosed by muscle biopsy.

Ring fibres: characteristic of myotonic dystrophy, but found less commonly in many other neuromuscular disorders, especially other myopathies. Ring fibres represent fibres in which several myofibrils have become displaced, after disruption, from their normal longitudinal alignment and have taken up a spiral location around the edge of the fibre. This change in location indicates the fluidity of the sarcoplasm in muscle fibres at body temperature.

Sarcoplasmic masses: in myotonic dystrophy peripherally located zones of sarcoplasm devoid of myofibrils but containing ribosomes and tubules may be seen. In some cases most of the fibres in the biopsy may show this change.

Fibre splitting: a feature of chronic myopathic or neurogenic disorders. In the latter it is characteristically found in hypertrophied Type 1 fibres.

Muscle spindles: show a characteristic abnormality in myotonic dystrophy, in which the intrafusal muscle fibres show splitting and proliferation.

Hyaline fibres: Duchenne muscular dystrophy, particularly in the early stages. Rare in other muscular dystrophies, but a few hyaline fibres are often seen in limb–girdle dystrophy.

Moth-eaten fibres: disruption and distortion of the intermyofibrillar network, often with a whorled appearance, best seen in NADH preparations. A non-specific change particularly prominent in inflammatory myopathy.

11.5   Relation of pathological change to clinical disability or stage of disorder

The degree of pathological change in a muscle biopsy in any disorder varies, not only with the degree of disability of the patient as a whole, a factor reflecting the stage of the disease at which the biopsy is taken, but with the rate of progression or healing, and with the degree of involvement of the muscle biopsied. The latter is particularly important since a biopsy of a clinically normal muscle may show marked abnormalities in many myopathies, especially in metabolic myopathies. It is therefore difficult to suggest a prognosis from study of a single muscle biopsy in myopathic disorders. In the muscular dystrophies different muscles show different degrees of involvement at any given time. For example the legs are relatively spared in facio-scapulo-humeral muscular dystrophy, but more severely involved than the arms in the early stages of Duchenne muscular dystrophy. In some neurogenic disorders, however, prominent fibre-type grouping may be found in muscles of virtually normal strength and bulk implying a relatively slow progression and effective reinnervation. This is especially typical of Type 3 or Type 4 spinal muscular atrophy, and of the neuronal form of Charcot–Marie–Tooth disease.

11.6 Are sequential biopsies useful?

Repeated muscle biopsies rarely provide useful information in assessing prognosis. The outcome is usually more accurately predictable from clinical observation. However, repeated biopsy may be useful in assessing the effect of treatment in inflammatory myopathy, and perhaps in certain metabolic myopathies. In inflammatory myopathy the development of steroid myopathy is a particular hazard of management and needle biopsy of the quadriceps muscle is useful in assessing the activity of the disease and the development of this complication.

Muscle biopsy is also sometimes used in family studies of patients with genetic myopathies. Generally, blood creatine kinase estimations are more useful in assessing carrier status or the presence of disease in families with muscular dystrophies, but in families with disorders not usually associated with a raised CK level, e.g. nemaline myopathy or central core disease, muscle biopsy may be useful as a method for acquiring information for genetic counselling. In genetic neurogenic conditions EMG is a more useful screening procedure than muscle biopsy.

Index

199

Printed in the United States
By Bookmasters